AVOCATIONAL ACTIVITIES FOR THE HANDICAPPED

All of the activities are classified and coded according to the complete classification of avocational activities previously developed by the senior author.

Readers are not expected to agree with all of the authors' impressions of activities. The Handbook has been planned to be provocative and controversial to stimulate counselors, whether they agree with the descriptions in the book or not, to think in new ways about the psychological and sociological framework within which activities are pursued.

Special features include:

CHECK LIST of environmental factors associated with the activity. Does it require much space or equipment?

CHECK LIST of social-psychological factors in an activity. Is it aesthetic or utilitarian? Creative or pre-patterned? Abstract or concrete?

CODED IMPAIRMENT TABLES to show whether a person with a certain type impairment would perform the activity. Could a blind person do this without help? Could a person do it if the rules were modified or special equipment were provided?

ENERGY OUTPUT TABLES for use with people having severe systemic impairments, especially heart patients. All of the activities are rated in terms of energy output ranging, for example, from 2 mets in playing cards to a range of 10 to 26 mets for wrestling.

QUICK FIND LIST at the end of the Handbook to help the reader to quickly locate all of the activities suitable for an individual with a particular impairment.

LIBRARY CLASSIFICATION NUMBERS for Dewey Decimal and Library of Congress systems. The reader who wants further information goes directly to the shelves without having to look up the location in a card catalog.

The descriptions of the avocational activities in this handbook are written for the person searching for an avocational activity. The Handbook is designed for use in avocational counseling by counselors, recreation therapists, occupational therapists and social workers.

Each activity is sufficiently described so that a preliminary decision can be made as to whether a given activity is suitable for a specific individual. The narratives emphasize the phenomenological and other psychological dimensions of the activity and also describe the interpersonal relationships and social settings of the activity.

Publication Number 922

AMERICAN LECTURE SERIES

A Publication in

The BANNERSTONE DIVISION *of*

AMERICAN LECTURES IN SOCIAL AND REHABILITATION PSYCHOLOGY

Editors of the Series

JOHN G. CULL, PH.D.
Director, Regional Counselor Training Program
Department of Rehabilitation Counseling
Virginia Commonwealth University
Fishersville, Virginia

and

RICHARD E. HARDY, ED.D.
Chairman, Department of Rehabilitation Counseling
Virginia Commonwealth University
Richmond, Virginia

The American Lecture Series in Social and Rehabilitation Psychology offers books which are concerned with man's role in his milieu. Emphasis is placed on how this role can be made more effective in a time of social conflict and a deteriorating physical environment. The books are oriented toward descriptions of what future roles should be and are not concerned exclusively with the delineation and definition of contemporary behavior. Contributors are concerned to a considerable extent with prediction through the use of a functional view of man as opposed to a descriptive, anatomical point of view.

Books in this series are written mainly for the professional practitioner; however, academicians will find them of considerable value in both undergraduate and graduate courses in the helping services.

Avocational Activities for the Handicapped

A Handbook for Avocational Counseling

By

ROBERT P. OVERS, Ph.D.
Research Coordinator
Curative Workshop of Milwaukee

ELIZABETH O'CONNOR

and

BARBARA DEMARCO

With a Foreword by

George T. Wilson, Re.D.
Assistant Superintendent of Schools
Division of Municipal Recreation and
Adult Education
Milwaukee, Wisconsin

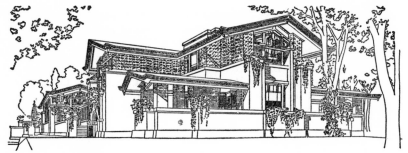

CHARLES C THOMAS · PUBLISHER
Springfield · Illinois · U.S.A.

Published and Distributed Throughout the World by
CHARLES C THOMAS • PUBLISHER
Bannerstone House
301-327 East Lawrence Avenue, Springfield, Illinois, U.S.A.

© *1974, by* CHARLES C THOMAS • PUBLISHER
ISBN 0-398-02975-X
Library of Congress Catalog Card Number: 73-11104

Printed in the United States of America
N-1

Library of Congress Cataloging in Publication Data

Overs, Robert P
    Avocational activities for the handicapped.

(American lecture series, publication no. 922. A publication in the Bannerstone division of American lectures in social and rehabilitation psychology)
    Includes bibliographical references.
    1. Rehabilitation counseling—Handbooks, manuals, etc. 2. Handicapped—Recreation—Handbooks, manuals, etc. I. O'Conner, Elizabeth, joint author. II. Demarco, Barbara, joint author. III. Title. [DNLM: 1. Counseling. 2. Handicapped. 3. Leisure activities. QT250 096a 1973]
HD7255.5.093   362'.0425   73-11104
ISBN 0-398-02975-X

EDITORS' FOREWORD

As a result of the Protestant work ethic it is quite natural that vocational counseling had to become a well established, recognized discipline before the concept of avocational counseling was accepted. However, as a result of technological changes and many other alterations in our life style, the effective and intelligent use of leisure time is becoming of prime concern and is moving up the hierarchy of national priorities. There have been a few other books published in the area of avocational counseling; however, we feel this one will become a landmark publication in that it provides avocational counseling information for many individuals who have leisure time but for whom avocational activities have not been too readily accessible in the past.

This outstanding text offers the recreational practitioner material which will enhance his effectiveness in providing avocational counseling to those with various disabilities. The book is organized in a way which makes it readily usable by professional practitioners. Since it is practitioner oriented and directed toward improving the quality of life for disabled persons. We are pleased to have this book appear in the *Social and Rehabilitation Psychology Series.*

Stuarts Draft, Va.
1974

JOHN G. CULL, PH.D.
RICHARD E. HARDY, ED.D.
Consulting Editors

The following books have appeared thus far in the Social and Rehabilitation Psychology Series:

VOCATIONAL REHABILITATION: PROFESSION AND PROCESS
John G. Cull and Richard E. Hardy

CONTEMPORARY FIELD WORK PRACTICES IN REHABILITATION
John G. Cull and Craig R. Colvin

SOCIAL AND REHABILITATION SERVICES FOR THE BLIND
Richard E. Hardy and John G. Cull

FUNDAMENTALS OF CRIMINAL BEHAVIOR AND CORRECTIONAL SYSTEMS
John G. Cull and Richard E. Hardy

MEDICAL AND PSYCHOLOGICAL ASPECTS OF DISABILITY
A. Beatrix Cobb

DRUG DEPENDENCE AND REHABILITATION APPROACHES
Richard E. Hardy and John G. Cull

INTRODUCTION TO CORRECTIONAL REHABILITATION
Richard E. Hardy and John G. Cull

VOLUNTEERISM: AN EMERGING PROFESSION
John G. Cull and Richard E. Hardy

APPLIED VOLUNTEERISM IN COMMUNITY DEVELOPMENT
Richard E. Hardy and John G. Cull

VOCATIONAL EVALUATION FOR REHABILITATION SERVICES
Richard E. Hardy and John G. Cull

ADJUSTMENT TO WORK: A GOAL OF REHABILITATION
John G. Cull and Richard E. Hardy

SPECIAL PROBLEMS IN REHABILITATION
A. Beatrix Cobb

FOREWORD

THE NEW LEISURE ETHIC suggests that the old concept of expressions of life style in terms of isolated blocks of time for work, play and meeting creature comfort needs, with each time block shifting in response to individual circumstances, may be undergoing a substantial change. Rather than filling time slots and assuming that each starts with potential boredom, the leisure ethic focuses on a developmental activity continuum expressive of man's quest for the uniqueness of his human dignity, concern for the quality of life and attainment of maximum potential.

The senseless search for material success at any cost and, often, when attained, the further pursuit of escape routes through drugs, fantasy and noise, lead only to the realization that the individual's personality has been destroyed. Man's value judgments may have to change so work, play, education and creature comfort demands can blend harmoniously into a positive life style. The freedom of the will and true self realization demand controls from within as well as externally in the pursuit of happiness.

There is little doubt that the significance of leisure whether expressed in terms of time slots or the new ethic is increasing in importance. A process by which this design for leisure will largely be met in the future is avocational counseling. The major tool of avocational counseling is the computer; its substance is a model consisting of an interest finder and resource inventory. Its special expertise is the warm human element of an understanding counselor. The goal is self-discovery, development of potential and an improved quality of life. Avocational counseling functions: to open doors for those in the mainstream of life through a maze of locally available outlets; to assist those on the fringe of the mainstream limited by physical, mental or cultural deprivation; and to ease the transition of the sheltered to return to the mainstream.

This book is on the cutting edge of new and significant development in the realm of leisure services. Avocational counseling will surely become as commonplace in the future as are parks, playgrounds and recreation centers today.

GEORGE T. WILSON, RE.D.
Assistant Superintendent of Schools
Division of Municipal Recreation
    and Adult Education
Milwaukee, Wisconsin

PREFACE

THIS IS THE THIRD PUBLICATION in a series of works designed to bring to the field of avocational counseling tools and techniques comparable to those developed in vocational counseling. The first step was the construction of an avocational activities classification and coding system. This was published as part of the MILWAUKEE MEDIA FOR REHABILITATION RESEARCH REPORTS series under the title "Avocational Activities Inventory" No. 5, June 1968. It was revised in November 1971 and became No. 5A.[1]

The "Avocational Activities Inventory" contains a comprehensive classification and numerical code for nearly all avocational activities. A set of "Avocational Activities File Labels" issued in April 1972 as No. 5C using the same classification and coding system was constructed to simplify setting up a vertical file to hold information about avocational activities.[2]

The present book presents descriptive narratives and other pertinent information about a selected group of avocations. The avocations included are classified and coded according to the classification system in the "Avocational Activities Inventory."

---

[1]"Avocational Activities Inventory," rev. ed., Report No. 5A (November, 1971). Part of *Milwaukee Media for Rehabilitation Research Reports* series, Research Department, Curative Workshop of Milwaukee, Milwaukee, Wisconsin.

[2]"Avocational Activities File Labels, Report No. 5C (April, 1972). Part of *Milwaukee Media for Rehabilitation Research Reports* series, Research Department, Curative Workshop of Milwaukee, Milwaukee, Wisconsin.

ACKNOWLEDGMENTS

THE PRESENT VOLUME is based on research and development done under contract with the United States Office of Education, Project Number NO. 59-2728 (1-D-055). We are grateful to the Office of Education for the support without which this work could not have been undertaken. Contractors undertaking such projects under Government sponsorship are encouraged to express freely their professional judgment in the conduct of the project. Points of view or opinions stated do not, therefore, necessarily represent official Office of Education position or policy.

The overall model for the work was the extraordinarily useful classification system, the *Dictionary of Occupational Titles*.[3]

Staff members of the Research Department of the Curative Workshop made the following contributions. In addition to the authors, Greg Houghton, Michael Santovec, Angela Varela, and David Wiemer wrote some of the activity descriptions. Barbara Olszweski, R.P.T., helped with the impairment coding. Mary Zolnowski classified the activities by the Dewey Decimal and Library of Congress codes. Maxine Schuldt, R.P.T. Coordinator of Physical Restoration, Darlene Rose, former Supervisor of the Speech Department, and Arlene Murry, O.T.R. Clinical Supervisor helped in developing the impairment code. Kathy McCormick, R.P.T. and Mary Beth Petersen, R.N. independently made preliminary ratings of activities with the impairment code.

Madalyn Braun, Supervisor of the Low Vision Clinic reviewed impairment ratings for the blind and low vision impairments. Bonnie Weissenfluh, Supervisor, Speech and Hearing Dept., reviewed the ratings for the hearing, speech and aphasia categories. George Hellmuth, M.D., cardiologist and Director of the Cardiac Work Classification Unit of the Curative Workshop furnished

---

[3]U.S. Dept. of Labor, *Dictionary of Occupational Titles* 3rd ed. (Washington, D.C., Govt. Printing Office) Vols. I and II 1965 and Supplement 1966.

background information for the reporting of energy output in METS, reviewed the assignment of energy expenditure require-ments for each activity and set up a model for assigning energy output limits for class III and class IV heart cases.

Corrine Aiholzer, O.T.R. Supervisor, Occupational Therapy Dept., Arlene Murray O.T.R., Clinical Supervisor, Linda Lynkie-wicz, O.T.R. Supervisor, Home Service Occupational Therapy Dept., Rosemary Rinzel, O.T.R. and Annette Christensen, O.T.R,. working as a team, reviewed all other impairment ratings.

Helen Christenson, Librarian, Chief of Processing, Milwaukee Public Library advised on the use of the Dewey Decimal and Library of Congress coding systems. Other library staff members were most helpful in facilitating the library research. William Hillman, Program Specialist, Bureau of Education for the Handi-capped, U. S. Office of Education helped with advice and en-couragement.

We are thankful to many other friends too numerous to mention who reviewed preliminary drafts of narratives and made suggestions about avocational activities with which they were familiar. Our specific debt to the existing literature on avoca-tional activities is to be found in footnotes where specific infor-mation was cited. Our general debt is too extensive to record.

INTRODUCTION

THE DESCRIPTIONS IN THIS BOOK are written from the point of view of a person searching for an avocational activity and are designed for use in avocational counseling by counselors, recreation therapists, occupational therapists, and social workers. During the rest of this introduction these four professions will be referred to under the term "counselor(s)" used generically. The descriptions attempt to tell enough about each activity so that a preliminary decision may be made as to whether a given activity is suitable for a special individual.

In contrast to most textbooks and other literature in the field of recreation, this volume is not written from the point of view of the program developer or recreation leader. It does not attempt to give all of the information necessary to set up and supervise an activity. For instance, detailed game rules are usually omitted. The emphasis in the narrative is on the phenomenological and other psychological dimensions of the activity, the interpersonal relationships involved and the social setting in which it occurs.

For a number of reasons, the same amount of space is not given each category. Partly this was because it was easier to obtain materials on some activities than on others. However, an effort was made to explore as many ramifications as possible of such commonplace activities as television watching and radio listening because of the importance of these activities in the lives of the homebound disabled.

There was a continuing editorial problem of balancing comprehensiveness of coverage with more intensive coverage of a particular activity. As an example, Slovenko and Knight, in their fascinating book, *Motivations in Play, Games and Sports* devoted nineteen pages to dancing, seven pages to chess and eighteen pages to baseball. With our coverage of a wider range of avocational activities, treating each activity this intensively, much as we should have liked to do so, would have led to an encyclopedia far beyond the reach of our time and money resources.[4]

Most of the narratives were written by the three authors. No effort was made to develop a uniform writing style. It was felt that a variety of styles would better maintain reader interest. Although a considerable amount of factual material has been included in the narratives, much of the material is subjective and impressionistic. It is not expected that readers will agree with all of our impressions of activities. We planned to be provocative and controversial to stimulate counselors, whether they agreed with us or not, to think in new ways about the psychological and sociological framework within which activities are pursued.

Information about avocational activities is presented in two ways. A check list section includes a listing of the environmental factors and social-psychological factors associated with the activity. It estimates whether the activity is within the physical and/or mental capacity of an individual with a given type of impairment and it gives an estimated range of energy expenditure expressed in METS.

In most cases, the check lists were prepared for each of the two digit code groups (e.g., 130 Table and Board Games). Where the physical activity requirements were particularly diverse as in "Sports," check list sheets were prepared for each three digit code group (e.g., 221, bicycling, motorcycling, unicycling) .

The environmental, social-psychological factors, and impairment limitations were prepared for groups of similar avocations. However, out of these groups only a few narrative descriptions were included to illustrate representative avocations in each group. Consequently, the environmental, social-psychological, and impairment limitations presented apply to many avocations *in addition to* those described in the narratives. For instance, specific reference is made in the impairment limitation section to ways in which modification in avocational activities may be made to accommodate the impairment for avocations which are *not* described in the narratives.

The code numbers for the avocational activities described

---

[4]R. Slovenko and J.A. Knight Eds., *Motivations in Play, Games and Sports* (Springfield, Illinois, Charles C Thomas, Publisher, 1967) .

either in the check lists or the narratives are given at the top of each page.

Following the check list sheet, the activity is described in narrative form. The Dewey Decimal and Library of Congress code numbers are presented at the beginning of each narrative or at the beginning of the check list sheet.

DEWEY DECIMAL SYSTEM NUMBER(S) AND LIBRARY OF CONGRESS NUMBER(S): These are included to enable a reader who wants more information on the activity to go directly to the library shelves without having to first look up in the library card catalog the location of the materials on the activity. The reader is advised to find out under which cataloging system the library which he uses operates. In general, public libraries use the Dewey Decimal system. Many university libraries use the Library of Congress system. The classifications found in libraries will not always agree exactly with the classifications we have made because of normal differences in judgment among classifiers and because the size of the library usually determines how detailed a classification code is used.

THE ENVIRONMENTAL AND SOCIAL-PSYCHOLOGICAL FACTORS involved in the group of activities for which representative narratives have been written are defined in the glossary further on in the Introduction.

IMPAIRMENT LIMITATIONS: Each type of impairment is coded in terms of whether or not the impairment will permit the activity to be carried on. The codes used are shown under abbreviations at the end of this section.

In general, the emphasis is on the impairment rather than on the demands of the activity. This is different from the system used by the *Dictionary of Occupational Titles* and other works. Our rationale is that occupational demands cannot ordinarily be altered greatly to meet the limitations caused by the client's impairments. However, in avocational activities, the activities usually can be altered to some degree to fit the limitations of the impaired persons because in general no minimum level of excellence has to be met. Social expectations and safety factors dictate some exceptions to this.

A classification of psycho-social impairments was omitted because there is so much variation between patients with the same diagnosis in their capacity for participating in any given activity. A variable in the rating of the *blind* is at what point in time the impairment occurred. Thus, the recently blinded have a large store of information and may not need new information input in order to carry on an activity.

With respect to the classification of *retardation,* we have limited our analysis to the educable retarded (mild, IQ 50 to 70).[5] Our analysis makes no effort to classify the activities in terms of the capacities of the trainable retarded (moderate, IQ 35 to 50), the severe (IQ 20 to 35) or the profound (IQ under 20).

The recommended energy expenditure limits for classes of organic heart disease are as follows. These are given in calories which are expressed as a measurement in terms of METS.[6]

Class	Severity Level	Expenditure Limits Permitted
I	prime (none)	Over 7 calories/min.
I	minimal	Energy expenditure continuous up to 5 calories/min., intermittent up to 6.6 calories/min.
II	moderate	Energy expenditure continuous up to 2.5 calories/min., intermittent up to 4 calories/min.
III	severe	Energy expenditure continuous up to 2 calories/min., intermittent up to 2.7 calories/min.
IV	very severe	Energy expenditure up to 1.5 calories/min.

ENERGY EXPENDITURE: The energy expenditure has been estimated for each of the avocational activities. It is measured in a unit called the MET. One MET is the amount of energy expended while resting and it is equivalent to an oxygen consumption of 250 ml/min. or 1 calorie. A MET includes the amount of

[5]Rick Heber, *A Manual on Terminology and Classification in Mental Retardation,* monograph supplement to *American Journal of Mental Deficiency* Albany.

[6]George Hellmuth, M.D. Adapted from "Work and Heart Disease in Wisconsin," *Journal of the American Medical Association,* Vol. 198, (December 26, 1966), pp. 133-37, which in turn is adopted with revisions from the American Heart Association and the American Medical Association, Committee on Medical Rating of Physical Impairments.

energy which is expended on the metabolic level in relationship to the energy expended in performing the activity. A MET therefore is a more accurate measurement of the total energy expenditure. For example, a person playing cards is using about twice as much energy as he would use if he were sleeping. His energy expenditure in METS would be 2.0. This is based on information summarized from the professional literature by cardiologist George Hellmuth, M.D., primarily from "Physiological Effect of Work on the Heart" by Lucien Broauha, appearing in Warshaw, Leon J. (ed.), *The Heart in Industry*, Paul B. Hoeber, Inc., Medical Division of Harper and Brothers, 1960.

The impairment limitation *seizures* as used here is defined as applying to individuals who actually suffer seizures. Individuals whose potential seizures are adequately controlled by medication may, pursuant to their physician's advice, not be limited in the ways we have indicated under seizures.

In our opinion, all ratings of impairment limitations are somewhat relative. Events can happen anywhere, even in the course of daily living at home. An *uncontrolled epileptic* can be injured in a fall regardless of where he is or what he is doing. Therefore our ratings assume that the activity is not hazard-free but merely that it entails no more hazard than would be normally encountered if the participant were pursuing a normal round of non-institutional living.

The classification of *aphasia* was very gross. There was no attempt to distinguish between aphasia for oral communication as against aphasia for written language.

The activities believed possible in spite of the aphasia were rated without taking into consideration that aphasia is characteristically associated with stroke which in turn is found with much higher frequency in middle and old age, all of which make it unlikely that because of his general physical condition the aphasic individual could participate in moderate to strenuous physical activities even though the aphasia itself was not an obstacle to this.

Just as with the blind, what the aphasic can do depends in part on the store of information which he had available prior to the onset of the impairment. Thus he may already know game rules so that the impairment of the receptive ability may not be as limiting as it otherwise might be.

The *hands impaired* category is complicated by the fact that some impaired individuals learn to manipulate pencils, paint brushes, punch sticks, and other devices with their mouths and head movements to do many of the things other people do with their hands. Thus, for this type of impairment there is a wide range of achievement depending upon individual training, equipment, and motivation.

For the activities of reaching, fingering, handling, feeling, stooping, kneeling, crouching, and crawling, the definitions published in the *Dictionary of Occupational Titles* were used.[7]

The respiratory impairment category includes not only avoiding the environmental conditions listed under Fumes, Odors, Toxic Conditions, Dust, and Poor Ventilation in the *Dictionary of Occupational Titles,* but also respiratory deficiencies which limit the impaired person's energy output expenditure.

All of the classifications discussed above postulate an average range of human behavior and consequently classification judgments are made in terms of an average individual carrying on the activity in an average way in an average situation. It is easy to point out exceptions to this classification schema, as it is with most other classification systems.

Naturally, in the case of certain severe impairments, the individual should check with his physician when there is any doubt as to whether participating in the activity could result in an accident or further impairment. This is of special concern in the case of advanced impairments, especially Class III and IV heart cases and severe respiratory impairments.

The information and recommendations contained in this publication have been compiled from sources believed to be reliable and to represent the best current opinion on the subject. No warranty, guarantee, or representation is made by the authors as to the absolute correctness or sufficiency of any representation in connection therewith; nor can it be assumed that all acceptable

---

[7]U.S. Dept. of Labor, *Dictionary of Occupational Titles,* Vol. 2, 3rd ed., (Washington, D.C., Govt. Printing Office) , p. 655.

safety measures are contained in this publication nor that other or additional measures may not be required under certain conditions or circumstances.

Originally it had been hoped to have each activity judged in terms of its feasibility for each type of impairment limitation and to report the degree of reliability among judges. The editorial problems in trying to make this as comprehensive as possible led us to group together activities into categories so broad that low reliability among judges resulted.

As the next best available control the following judging or rating procedure was used. The initial ratings were made by the senior author, a counseling psychologist with extensive experience in vocational counseling with the disabled, and by a physical therapist.

An experienced counselor for the blind in a low vision clinic, herself legally blind, reviewed the ratings on the blind and low vision impairments categories. A speech therapy department supervisor reviewed the ratings for the hearing, speech and aphasia categories. A nationally known cardiologist reviewed the energy expenditure requirements for each activity.

Two supervisors of occupational therapy departments working with a team of three other OTR's reviewed all of the impairment ratings not reviewed by the specialists indicated above. Differences of opinion among judges were resolved by discussion, usually resulting in suggesting how an activity could be pursued with suitable modifications.

The ratings presented then represent the result of careful judgments by knowledgeable professionals. They may be regarded as exploratory guidelines against which each counselor using this book may check his own judgment. They do not offer the degree of assurance which a high measured reliability among judges would give us and further work in this direction is desirable.

ABBREVIATIONS

DD   Dewey Decimal System Library classification system number

LC   Library of Congress classification system number

METS Energy expenditure unit (amount of energy expended while resting and is equivalent to an oxygen consumption of 250 ml/min. or 1 calorie)

+   The activity can be performed by an individual with the impairment.

O   The activity cannot be performed by an individual with the impairment.

M   The activity can be performed in spite of the impairment, provided appropriate modifications in the activity are made. This may include such things as changing game rules, providing additional tools, jigs, and fixtures, or providing help by other people.

S   Some but not all of the activities can be performed by an individual with the impairment.

GLOSSARY OF TERMS

Environmental Factors

N o specific environment: surrounding conditions neither influence nor modify ability to practice activity.

Specialized environment and/or climate: surroundings must satisfy certain requirements inherent in the nature of the activity, e.g., snow, ice, or water required.

Modicum of space: activity is not severely hampered by space limitations.

Unlimited spaces: activity requires extensive use of space.

Requires little or no equipment: the extent or expense of material goods to be acquired in order to partake in the activity is so negligible as to be a minor factor in considering the suitability of the activity to a client. Generally less than $10.00.

Equipment a major factor: outlay for additional equipment is extensive or expensive enough to constitute a major factor in considering the suitability of the activity to a client. Generally more than $10.00. Includes the cost of supplies if these are expensive.

Equipment normally at hand: while there may be a number of materials required, their nature is such that they are usually included in a list of household items. Or, materials can be easily obtained, e.g., by particular service organizations (public library). Includes easily accessible public or semipublic playing courts for tennis, handball, etc.

Equipment not necessarily at hand: items are less commonly owned, more often purchased, rented, or borrowed, e.g., sewing machine.

Social-Psychological Factors

AESTHETIC: activity appeals to subjective appreciation of beauty, or appreciation of the activity for itself rather than for possible results or practical applications.

UTILITARIAN: activity pursued for its practical, serviceable aspects, or activity directed towards specific goal achievement.

CREATIVE: activity lends itself to imaginative variations or innovations.

PRE-PATTERNED: the outcome of the activity is already determined by some set standards; individual variations are minimal.

ABSTRACT: activity involves thought process of which there is no tangible evidence.

CONCRETE: activity has specific applications, or is experienced in immediate, physical, tangible results.

GROUP EFFORT: activity allows for or requires cooperative work of two or more. Includes games or sports with two or more participants on a team.

INDIVIDUAL EFFORT: activity is dependent upon the efforts of one person only.

STRUCTURED: results of activity somewhat limited by predetermined standards of expectations. Includes game and sports rules.

UNSTRUCTURED: activity encourages unlimited creativity, imagination, and initiative.

SUPERVISED: activity presided over by some regulatory force, person or rule system, which makes certain demands and controls participation in the activity. Includes rules of games and sports.

UNSUPERVISED: the manner in which the activity is pursued or practiced is determined by the individual or sets of individuals involved.

OPPORTUNITY FOR RECOGNITION: successful participation in the activity results in positive reinforcement in the form of praise, awards, expressed admiration, etc.

LITTLE OPPORTUNITY FOR RECOGNITION: results of the activity important to or noticed by only the individual; little outside reinforcement.

HOW TO USE THE QUICK FIND LIST

IN THE QUICK FIND list under each environmental factor, social-psychological factor and impairment and energy expenditure range are listed the codes for the avocational activities in which these factors and impairments are relevant.

Only the impairments coded + (can do), M (can do with modifications), and S (can do some of the activities) are listed. The categories coded O (cannot do) were omitted from the QUICK FIND list as it is designed to help find things the impaired can do, not what they cannot do.

To save space, the numbered code was used rather than classification titles, although admittedly this is hard on the reader. The code numbers were used instead of page numbers because the counselor who uses the QUICK FIND list regularly will soon memorize the code numbers as they relate to named categories.

The QUICK FIND list is used in this way: if it is desired to find all of the activities which are associated with a specific environmental factor, a specific social-psychological factor, can be pursued with a particular impairment limitation, or fall within a specific energy expenditure range, the pertinent factor is located on the QUICK FIND list. The reader then scans through the book following the code numbers listed on the QUICK FIND list.

To locate activities which an individual with a specific impairment can do, first go through the list marked + (can do). If nothing suitable is found, then go through the list marked S (can do some of the activities). If no appropriate activity is found there, go through the list marked M (can do with modifications). If you still don't find anything you're on your own (we've done our best!).

CONTENTS

**Avocational Activities
for the Handicapped**

Avocational Activities for the Handicapped

100 Games

The large numbers of games available has made it impossible to offer comprehensive coverage of this major category of activities. Accordingly, we have described only a few games for illustrative purposes. For exhaustive listings, the reader will need to consult listings of commercial games publishers.

112 Throwing Games, e.g., catch, frisbie, keep-away, pig-in-the-middle, etc.

ENVIRONMENTAL FACTORS: indoor, outdoor, no specific environment, unlimited space, requires little or no equipment, equipment not necessarily at hand.

SOCIAL-PSYCHOLOGICAL FACTORS: aesthetic, pre-patterned, concrete, group effort, individual effort, structured, unsupervised, opportunity for recognition.

Impairment Limitations

blind	M1	balance	S1	*hands impaired*	1	2
low vision	M1	seizures	+	reaching	+	0
hearing	+	*aphasia:*		handling	+	0
speech	+	receptive	+	fingering	+	0
retardation	+	expressive	+	feeling	+	0
memory	+	mixed	+	no hands	0	
impaired:						
stooping	M2	wheel chair	M2	bed patient	0	
kneeling	M2	semi-ambulant	S1	respiratory	0	
crouching	M2	Class III heart	0	*Energy Expenditure in*		
crawling	+	Class IV heart	0	*METS:* 4-8		

M1 use easily grasped soft objects like bean bags
M2 need companion to pick up object if it drops
S1 may play if sitting down or holding on

Throwing games involve the use of an object—ball, frisbie, or on the *very* spontaneous level, someone's hat—which the players toss back and forth. Usually this is a cooperative venture, engaged in for the sheer joy of the sport and/or as a means of gaining skill in catching and throwing for use in other games like baseball.

Certain throwing games, e.g., keep-away and pig-in-the-middle, introduce elements of competition. In an informal way, they are versions of some far more sophisticated games like football: the idea of these games is for one team to maintain control of the ball (or whatever) while the other team is trying to capture it. Pig-in-the-middle is a three-player version: two "catchers" throw the ball back and forth until the third manages to intercept its flight; he then becomes a catcher, while the player who would have caught the ball if it had not been intercepted becomes the "pig-in-the-middle." When more than three are playing, teams are formed, and one team tries to "keep away" from the other.

Like running games, throwing games require space; played indoors in close quarters, they pose a considerable danger to lamps, pictures, and other furnishings.

120 Target and Skill Games

ENVIRONMENTAL FACTORS: indoor, no specific environment, modicum of space, equipment a major factor, equipment not necessarily at hand.

SOCIAL-PSYCHOLOGICAL FACTORS: aesthetic, pre-patterned, concrete, individual effort, structured, supervised, opportunity for recognition, utilitarian.

Impairment Limitations

blind	0	balance	M2	*hands impaired:*	*1*	*2*
low vision	M1	seizures	+	reaching	M3	0
hearing	+	*aphasia:*		handling	M3	0
speech	+	receptive	+	fingering	M3	M3
retardation	+	expressive	+	feeling	M3	M3
memory	+	mixed	+	no hands	0	

impaired:					
stooping	M4	wheel chair	M4	bed patient	M6
kneeling	M4	semi-ambulant	M4	respiratory	M5
crouching	M4	Class III heart	M5	*Energy Expenditure in*	
crawling	+	Class IV heart	M6	*METS:* 1.6–5	

M1 limited to close up action like pickup sticks and tiddly winks
M2 if sitting or otherwise supported

M3 can manipulate games requiring only one hand but not those like pool, requiring two
M4 needs companion to pick up horseshoe, bean bags, etc.
M5 can do everything except possibly horseshoes but at a slower pace and for a shorter time
M6 keep to limited energy output games such as pickup sticks and tiddly winks

Many of the games in this general category are games which test physical dexterity but do not demand great physical exertion. In this, they can be used to advantage for those who cannot participate in strenuous recreation. Mental ability as well as physical dexterity is used in these games. Much of it is problem-solving—how to get out of a particular game situation. The solution rests in evaluation and response. Playing technique and luck combine to determine the outcome of the game. This puts the player in active and passive roles and tests his reaction to each. An important element of the games in categories 123 and 124 is that of competition. Satisfaction in playing is as much the result of outmaneuvering the opponent as it is pride in the evidence of physical and mental skills.

123 Darts

Darts, in contrast to many of the related throwing-at-target games has less bending over to pick things up which is an advantage for people who because of poor balance, poor coordination or lower extremity impairments are handicapped in bending over. The few darts which do not stick in the board may be retrieved more easily if the dart board is placed over a table or bed. For safety, don't be a target; stand behind the player who is throwing!

123 Ring-Toss, Ringstack

Ringstack is a low-skill game requiring the placement of variously dimensioned colored rings on a tapered pole, the largest ring being placed on the bottom of the stack and the rest continuing upward in diminishing sizes. The stack is capped by a plastic screw-on ball.

Ringstack is an excellent device for developing sense (sight) discrimination. It is easy to complete by the trial-and-error method. It requires mobility and manual skills. The game can be played alone or with others. It is useful in providing additional sight, touch and kinesthetic sensory stimulation.

Some perseverance and a willingness to try different approaches is required if first attempts fail at hitting the right combination. The game teaches the player self-reliance and rewards him with a sense of accomplishment if successful. It is estimated that some individuals with one or more of the following impairments may successfully participate in the activity: audio impairments, cerebral palsy, mental retardation, Perthes disease and visual impairments.

The game can be adapted to a severely impaired cerebral palsied child by having the child indicate to the recreational therapist which ring to place on the stack.

123 Horseshoes LC: GV 1095

Horseshoes are pitched back and forth between two stakes set 40 feet apart, the object being to ring the stake with the horseshoe and if not, come as close as possible to the stake. The game can be played as singles between two players or as doubles between two teams of two players each.

Many families own sufficient land to make it possible to construct a court in their own back yard which is a great convenience over sports which require a great deal of travel to reach the place where the sport is carried out. This has the further advantage of a focus for neighborhood social interaction.

The sport is well adapted for a wide age span and for both sexes. Individuals with the use of only one arm may play it on an equal basis with the nonimpaired person.

123 Bean Bags

Bean bags is played by throwing ten cloth bags each full of beans through holes in a board set at a 45 degree angle with the floor with the lower end resting on the floor and the upper end supported by hinged wooden legs. There are five different sized holes in the board yielding scores of 5, 10, 15, 20, and 25. The smaller the hole, the larger the score.

Like horseshoes and darts, vertical as well as horizontal control is needed. There is much bending, stooping and kneeling to retrieve the bean bags many of which are recovered from under the bean bag board.

This game is well adapted to the living room, dining room or recreation room of the average sized house or apartment. It offers a great deal of practice in mental addition of fives and multiples of five.

124 Secondary Target Games

Secondary target games: games in which an object is propelled toward a target by means of a second object, e.g., pool, billiards, bumper pool, shuffleboard, marbles, tiddly winks, etc. DD: 794.6-.73. LC: GV 1099, GV 891-9.

Depending on whether the players consider games as recreation or as serious business, games in this category hold remarkable possibilities for social intercourse. Now, a *real* pool or billiard player is dead serious about his game, so these social possibilities will remain, for him, unexplored. His joy will come from knowing that he knows how to play his game and his satisfaction will derive from playing it. The movie "The Hustler" well illustrates the intensity of this kind of play. But that kind of devotion would seem to classify the game more as life's blood than as avocational activity.

By contrast, the prospect of a *real* tiddly wink player strikes one as rather ludicrous. Most people tend to dabble in these games, rather than pursue them as professions. It is this attitude towards games, that of the dilettante and not the devotee that suggests the added dimension of games as inducing social contacts. The players' very lack of intensity in play makes it possible for them to recognize other features of the game—its humorous or ridiculous sides. Mistakes, bad plays, bad luck are much easier pills to swallow when taken with a healthy sense of humor. The general hilarity that attends the more glaring errors adds a sense of spirit to the game that serious pursuit often kills. This lack of seriousness may, if extended further than some would wish, become irritating; on the other hand, there are occasions when humor is a definite requisite. Finding the right balance is the concern of the players involved.

130 Table and Board Games

ENVIRONMENTAL FACTORS: indoor, no specific environment, modicum of space, equipment a major factor, equipment not necessarily at hand.

SOCIAL-PSYCHOLOGICAL FACTORS: aesthetic, creative, pre-patterned, abstract, concrete, individual effort, structured, supervised, opportunity for recognition.

Impairment Limitations

blind	M1	balance	+	*hands impaired:*	*1*	*2*
low vision	+	seizures	+	reaching	+	M5
hearing	+	*aphasia:*		handling	+	M5
speech	+	receptive	M4	fingering	+	M5
retardation	M2	expressive	+	feeling	+	+
memory	M3	mixed	M4	no hands	M5	

impaired:

stooping	+	wheel chair	+	bed patient	+
kneeling	+	semi-ambulant	+	respiratory	+
crouching	+	Class III heart	+	*Energy Expenditure in*	
crawling	+	Class IV heart	+	*METS: 2—2.5*	

M1 use braille checker boards, dice, bingo, chess, etc., can do chinese checkers

M2 well suited for "work bench" game, have difficulty with chess

M3 well suited for "work bench" game, probably can do chinese checkers, have difficulty with monopoly, chess, etc.

M4 need visual clues

M5 may need adaptive device to move playing pieces around or a companion to move the pieces

Mentioned in this category are some of the games people play. It is theorized that playing games is parallel to coping with real-life anxieties.[8] The world, in play, is reduced to the area of the game. The situations encountered in games are paradigms of

[8]R. Slovenko and J. A. Knight, eds., *Motivations in Play, Games and Sports* (Springfield, Illinois, Charles C Thomas, 1967) p. 56.

confrontations within realistic social activities. Games challenge the player to creative responses in his attempt to master given situations. The player tries to make the best of his situation within the limits of the game rules. While skill is often an important factor in play, games are not solely a test of intellect. Games incorporate a social setting and the player's response to this is a test of emotional maturity. Enough social pressure can be exercised in a game to foster positive social behavior.

Games, as a gauge of emotional response, might be put to analytic or therapeutic use. That is, one might employ game-playing either to test the individual's emotional capacities or to correct or improve upon them or both. The games as categorized below stress different characteristics of play and call for different degrees or kinds of skills.

134 Money Games

Money games: games in which the goal is to acquire money, property, etc. DD: 793.5. LC: GV 1312.

These games allow the player to decide much for himself his course of play but also include the outside chance factor. That is, the player may decide the strategy he wants to pursue in order to become successful, but certain arbitrary factors of the game may interfere. For example, a player at Monopoly may decide to build up his property, but he may not land on the right places in time. Most often the games feature such contingencies and the player learns to be clever, resourceful and flexible. These games have instructive value. The player must learn to take calculated risks and to take the setbacks and disadvantages that ensue if his plans are frustrated. One might question the lesson of ruthless pursuit of one's own goal (opportunities to destroy one's opponent are especially evident in Monopoly). One might question also the goals so many of the games espouse, which deal primarily in economic gain and social status. As with the other games, there is as much to learn in losing as in winning, not only in terms of successful strategies, but also in terms of social behavior and coping with disappointments.

135 *Dual Combat Games*

Dual combat games: e.g., checkers, chess, Stratego, etc. DD: 794.1-.2. LC: GV 1313-1457, GV 1461-3.

These are games in which the level of play adjusts to the player's level of skill. That is, the games set up certain regulations of moves and an arbitrary goal. Within that framework, it is the players who determine the succession of moves and develop the strategies to achieve that set goal. Because the level of play is largely determined by the players and because there are only two players involved, it is important that the players be evenly matched. The game is frustrated if the competition offers too little or too great a challenge. This match between two players is important to the game in another way. These are games of aggression which, like many of the other games, arouse powerful emotions. When the game is only between two, the rivalry and possible hostility can become much more intense and intensely directed. Yet, games which demand concentrated mental effort demand also emotional control.

Checkers is dual combat at its most basic level. Checkers has been the format for many other dual combat games. Its simple rules and restricted game plan belie its strength. Checkers, played skillfully, can become a studied game of scientific play. Game play improves through practice. The uniformity of moves makes study of the game possible without a frustratingly complicated exercise of mental gymnastics.

Chess is believed to be the most popular game in the western world. Many more men than women play the game; it is a kind of surrogate warfare. The aggressive nature of the game is its most important characteristic. The object is to force the opposing king into a situation in which he must surrender: to do this, opposing defensive pieces are captured or intricate traps are laid for the king. One king is finally forced to admit defeat, even though he may be surrounded by his own defensive forces; this psychological-ly climactic moment of admitting defeat is frequently very intense.

Although the aggressive tendencies which are evident in chess are so important, players must sublimate them in order to play rationally. Chess carries with it a high degree of status, because both society and the players themselves are aware that competence in chess requires above average intelligence. But not even the most intelligent player can plan rationally if he is unable to keep his emotional responses under control. The chess player, therefore, must be able to deal with his own feelings as well as with the strengths of his opponent.

Individuals frequently play chess by telephone or mail, each player having a graphic model of the distribution of pieces. This type of play might be especially helpful for shut-ins; many prisons also run programs by which convicts are allowed to carry on such long-distance games with people outside the prison, providing both social contact and intellectual stimulation.

Stratego, though still a game of strategy, includes an additional factor—chance. The chance is taken when a player attacks a piece whose rank, because hidden, is unknown. This adds a surprise element to a game in which the player must have resource to strategic planning, cleverness, deception, foresight and a good memory. Unlike chess, in which all the possible outcomes of moves can be determined by mental exercise and careful scrutiny, Stratego makes use of suspense and hidden possibilities to effect an intriguing game.

140 Card Games

ENVIRONMENTAL FACTORS: indoor, no specific environment, modicum of space, requires little or no equipment, equipment normally at hand.

SOCIAL-PSYCHOLOGICAL FACTORS: aesthetic, pre-patterned, abstract, concrete, group effort, individual effort, structured, supervised, opportunity for recognition.

Impairment Limitations

blind	M1	balance	+	*hands impaired:*	*1*	*2*
low vision	M2	seizures	+	reaching	M5	M6
hearing	+	*aphasia:*		handling	M5	M6
speech	+	receptive	+	fingering	M5	M6
retardation	M3	expressive	+	feeling	+	+
memory	M4	mixed	+	no hands	M6	

impaired:

stooping	+	wheel chair	+	bed patient	+
kneeling	+	semi-ambulant	+	respiratory	+
crouching	+	Class III heart	+	*Energy Expenditure in*	
crawling	+	Class IV heart	+	*METS: 2–2.5*	

M1 Braille cards
M2 large print cards
M3 may manage simple games; probably have difficulty with bridge
M4 probably have difficulty with games like bridge or hearts where it is important to remember what cards other players hold; should be able to manage solitaire and cribbage
M5 may need card holder
M6 in addition to card holder, may need adaptive device or companion to manipulate cards

143 Games For Three or More, Playing as Individuals

Games for three or more, playing as individuals: e.g., poker, rummy, hearts, old maid, blackjack, canasta, seven card stud, etc. DD: 795.412. LC: GV 1295.C2, GV 1295.B, GV 1295.R8, GV 1251.3.

As the number of players in a card game increases, the importance of mutual consideration grows. While the players of a two-handed game may agree by unspoken mutual consent to play slowly and casually, in a larger game it is only courteous to pay fairly close attention to the cards. Within this framework, a group which plays together regularly will soon find an equilibrium point at which all players will be happy about the amount of social interaction and the amount of importance being attached to the game itself.

It is in these games that gambling takes on real importance. Many of them have little meaning if they aren't played *for* something, even if it be only matchsticks or plastic chips. The danger of an over-serious gambler upsetting the game is a real one; so are the problems of the poor loser and the individual who seems not to care whether he wins or not. If one player is on a winning streak, it will be noticed that other players tend either to band together against him or to lose interest in the game.

Many games are psychologically interesting in that the rules require that one player punish another. The game of "hearts" goes beyond this and sometimes requires a player to choose which player to punish. Even though it is only a game, there can be considerable emotional involvement in either giving out or receiving punishment.

In Blackjack each player attempts to collect cards which total as near 21 as possible without exceeding that number. Cards are dealt to the player one at a time until he feels that to accept one more card would mean exceeding 21. It is necessary to add and subtract fairly rapidly and this would indicate simple arithmetic skills. Five former patients who had suffered strokes were observed playing blackjack together. All performed the game well and no difference in arithmetic skills were noted. Each player quickly and correctly added his cards together and subtracted the sum from 21 and indicated whether he wanted more cards from the dealer.

144 *Games For Three or More, Playing as Teams*

Games for three or more, playing as teams: e.g., bridge, whist, sheepshead, pinochle, etc. DD: 795.416. LC: GV 1281, GV 1295.P6.

Games in which the players form teams are extremely popular. The immediate advantage to playing in teams, of course, is that it gives the player an ally with whom to contend against the other players. This can give the player a sense of security.

Partnerships often grow into lasting friendships which continue long after the bridge game is over. Husband-wife teams are common, but sometimes dangerous, since arguments about the game can carry over into other areas. It is important that partners not have skills which are quantitatively and qualitatively very different; if one partner begins to feel that he is carrying the team, the result can be disastrous to the players' friendship.

As in other card game situations, the attitude of the players towards the game is crucial. The player who makes too big a deal out of winning or losing spoils everyone's pleasure; worse still is the player who gets very upset about losing and then blames the loss on his partner's carelessness or lack of skill. Team games often do result in close friendships both within and among teams, and the kind of informal get-togethers that spring from "next week, our house," invitations.

150 Knowledge and Word Games

ENVIRONMENTAL FACTORS: indoor, no specific environment, modicum of space, requires little or no equipment, equipment normally at hand.

SOCIAL-PSYCHOLOGICAL FACTORS: aesthetic, creative, pre-patterned, abstract, group effort, individual effort, structured, unstructured, supervised, opportunity for recognition.

Impairment Limitations

blind	M1	balance	+	*hands impaired:*	*1*	*2*
low vision	+	seizures	+	reaching	+	M8
hearing	M2	*aphasia:*		handling	+	M8
speech	M3	receptive	M6	fingering	+	M8
retardation	M4	expressive	M7	feeling	+	+
memory	M5	mixed	0	no hands	M6	

impaired:

stooping	+	wheel chair	+	bed patient	+
kneeling	+	semi-ambulant	+	respiratory	+
crouching	+	Class III heart	+	*Energy Expenditure in*	
crawling	+	Class IV heart	+	*METS:* 2—2.5	

M1 use braille scrabble; probably can't do paper and pencil games, charades and memory games such as Brainstorm
M2 too slow at guessing games
M3 if stutters, write out answers to guessing games
M4 can simplify all of these games as appropriate
M5 probably can't do memory games
M6 simple paper and pencil games only
M7 nonverbal output games only
M8 will need adaptive device or assistant for paper and pencil games and Brainstorm

152 Guessing Games

Guessing games: e.g., 20 questions, I Spy, animal-vegetable-mineral, etc. DD: 793.73, 793.7. LC: PN 6366-6377.

Guessing games are good for large or small groups of any age.

There is a large variety of such games, running through a range of difficulty include games to fit the abilities of almost any group.

I Spy is an excellent example of this kind of game. Players choose an object which they hide after sending one player from the room. When this player returns, he begins to hunt for the hidden object. The others clap or sing or do both loudly when the hunter is near the hiding place; when he is a distance away from the object, the clapping and singing become soft. This continues until the hidden object is found.

I Spy is excellent for individuals with impaired receptive communication facility. They do not have to understand words and the game may be played even if the individual has some degree of hearing loss or even total vision loss. It is highly suitable for cross cultural interpersonal exchange where there is a language or concept barrier.

153 *Spelling Games*

Spelling games: e.g., Scrabble, Spill 'n' Spell, spelling bee, etc.

Spill 'n' Spell is a simple vocabulary game which incorporates much the same basic idea as Scrabble. Six former patients who had suffered strokes were observed as they performed Spill 'n' Spell. Scrabble had been tried previously and it was discovered that several of the patients had a great deal of difficulty with it. Accordingly, a simplified version of Spill 'n' Spell was substituted.

Procedure: The game is played by shaking approximately 18 dice out of a plastic cup. A letter is printed on each side of the dice (Braille markings may be made for blind or low vision). Each player tries to use the letters on the top side of the dice to form as many words as possible. Normally, players must form intersecting words, but in this case it was decided to allow the patients to form separated words. However, the ability to intersect words was considered to be evidence of a higher degree of skill in forming and using words. The total score for each turn is computed by squaring the total number of letters which the player used.

Six patients tried this game. The best player, on his first turn, used 12 letters, spelling three words of four letters apiece. He formed words rapidly and while the others were taking their turns, he quietly gave hints of possible words. On the second turn, he used 14 letters, spelling four words of six, three, three, and two letters and also formed a word seldom used, "cougar." He did not intersect any words, but this may be attributed to the fact that he took his turn first and thus did not gain much advantage from seeing other players form words.

The difference in performance in the next three players was slight. To rank the players, total score, the length of words, the ability to intersect words, the rapidity with which words were formed and the total number of letters used were all taken into account. The relative ranking of these players might easily be altered if different weight were given to different aspects of their performance.

The rate at which one patient formed various words was significantly reduced by what appeared to be sight impairments. Another patient needed a great deal of coaxing and encouragement even to complete words.

156 Memory Games

Memory games: e.g., Concentration, Brainstorm. DD: 793.735. LC: PN 6366-6377.

Brainstorm uses a regular deck of playing cards. The point of the game is to match cards of the same number which have been placed face down after having been seen once. The cards are deliberately placed in as spatially irregular a nonpattern as possible. Recall is entirely contingent on remembering the spatial arrangement of the cards. Five former patients who had suffered strokes were observed playing this game together. All had played cards for many years and all had played this game about two months before. After four complete games were played, the relative ability of each player was clearly established.

This game might be developed as a supplement to clinical tests of memory deficit.

160 Puzzles

Environmental factors: indoor, no specific environment, modicum of space, requires little or no equipment, equipment not necessarily at hand.

Social-psychological factors: aesthetic, pre-patterned, concrete, group effort, individual effort, structured, unsupervised, little opportunity for recognition.

Impairment Limitations

blind	S1	balance	+	*hands impaired:*	*1*	*2*
low vision	+	seizures	+	reaching	+	M1
hearing	+	*aphasia:*		handling	+	M1
speech	+	receptive	S5	fingering	+	M1
retardation	S2	expressive	S4	feeling	+	+
memory	S3	mixed	S5	no hands	M1	

impaired:

stooping	+	wheel chair	+	bed patient	+
kneeling	+	semi-ambulant	+	respiratory	+
crouching	+	Class III heart	+	*Energy Expenditure in*	
crawling	+	Class IV heart	+	*METS: 2.–2.5*	

M1 need device or assistant to help move pieces and write
S1 may do mental arithmetic puzzles and help on crosswords
S2 may do some of these at a simple level
S3 may have difficulty with those dependent on a retrievable fund of knowledge
S4 possible, if able to write
S5 jigsaw only

162 Crosswords, diacrostics, etc. DD: 793.732 LC: GV 1507.C7, PN 6369-6377

The person who is fascinated by words and the letters which build them will certainly find pleasure in working word puzzles—crosswords, diacrostics, anagrams, and the like. Puzzles like these cannot only challenge, but actually improve, one's knowledge of his native language.

The crossword is the most common, best known, and probably simplest of these word puzzles; although the format is simple, the puzzle itself may be quite complex and difficult. Other puzzles require doubling back and forth among steps. The anagram, for

example, calls for words to be formed by rearranging the letters
of other words. The puzzle may first call for a word of a certain
number of letters which fits a definition; to solve the anagram,
the letters of that word must then be rearranged.

Jigsaw puzzles require a flat surface, but word puzzles may be
solved almost anywhere: on a bus, train, or plane, in bed, or
curled up in an easy chair. Word puzzles make virtually no noise,
require little expenditure of physical energy, and an afficionado
may work them by the hour without suffering from boredom.
Word puzzles are an essentially solitary activity, but two people
may occasionally collaborate on one, and there is always the situation in which anyone who happens to be present is called on for
help, "Does anybody know a four-letter word for 'assistance'?"

170 Model Racing Games

ENVIRONMENTAL FACTORS: indoor, outdoor, modicum of space,
unlimited space, equipment a major factor, equipment not necessarily at hand.

SOCIAL-PSYCHOLOGICAL FACTORS: aesthetic, creative, pre-patterned, concrete, individual effort, structured, unsupervised, opportunity for recognition.

Impairment Limitations

				hands impaired:	1	2
blind	0	balance	S1			
low vision	+	seizures	+	reaching	M1	0
hearing	+	*aphasia:*		handling	M1	0
speech	+	receptive	+	fingering	M1	0
retardation	+	expressive	+	feeling	+	0
memory	+	mixed	+	no hands	0	

impaired:

stooping	S2	wheel chair	S2	bed patient	S3
kneeling	S2	semi-ambulant	S2	respiratory	+
crouching	S2	Class III heart	+	*Energy Expenditure in*	
crawling	+	Class IV heart	S3	*METS:* 2–4	

M1 could operate but not readily build models
S1 difficulty in controlling model airplanes in flight
S2 could operate cars and trains mounted on tables
S3 could assemble but not operate

The chief attraction of model racing games is that they are

helpful in propelling the player into a fantasy world in which his powers far exceed those he possesses in real life. The timid driver can send his model car skittering around a track at a speed which drivers of the Indianapolis 500 might envy, and the fellow who gets seasick in a row boat can sail his sloop to a victory at sea. Similarly, such activity can enable the ordinarily mild-mannered person to engage in a kind of cut-throat competition in which he would ordinarily never get involved. Competition in these games tends to be friendly but quite intense. Many enthusiasts enjoy building their own model or improving on the design and construction of models which they have purchased.

190 Miscellaneous Games

ENVIRONMENTAL FACTORS: indoor, no specific environment, modicum of space, equipment a major factor, equipment not necessarily at hand.

SOCIAL-PSYCHOLOGICAL FACTORS: aesthetic, utilitarian, creative, pre-patterned, abstract, concrete, group effort, individual effort, structured, unstructured, unsupervised, little opportunity for recognition.

Impairment Limitations

blind	M1	balance	+	*hands impaired:*	1	2
low vision	+	seizures	+	reaching	+	S4
hearing	+	*aphasia:*		handling	+	S4
speech	+	receptive	S2	fingering	+	S4
retardation	S1	expressive	S3	feeling	+	S4
memory	S1	mixed	S2	no hands	S4	

impaired:

stooping	+	wheel chair	+	bed patient	+
kneeling	+	semi-ambulant	+	respiratory	+
crouching	+	Class III heart	+	*Energy Expenditure in*	
crawling	+	Class IV heart	+	*METS:* 2–2.5	

M1 use Braille dominoes and dice
S1 dominoes and ouija
S2 dominoes, if rules are already known
S3 dominoes
S4 everything but ouija

191 *Dominoes* DD: 795.3 LC: GV 1467

The game is played with 28 dominoes. The object of the game is to attach a domino to the next domino which is only permitted if the attaching domino has the same number of spots. Points are made if the total number of spots at each end of the domino line add up to five or a multiple of five. The game is excellent for teaching very simple mental arithmetic. It may be played by two, three or four players.

192 *Computer Games* DD: 510.78 LC: QA 74, QA 76

There are, in general, two types of computer games. In the first kind, the computer acts as your opponent. Computers have been programmed to play a variety of games, varying from tic-tac-toe to chess. In this type of game you make a move and then the computer makes a move to counteract your move. The computer also acts as scorekeeper and provides a continuous printout of the status of the game.

In the second kind of game, the computer acts primarily as scorekeeper. This is very helpful in real-life simulation games (194) by permitting more complicated and more challenging situations. The computer evaluates your actions and projects their consequences on the current situation, thus updating the situations. Based on the results of your previous action, you can either continue or modify your strategy in obtaining the goal of the game. You may either play against other persons who are simultaneously taking actions which modify the current situation, or you may play a type of solitaire in which you attempt to solve a problem, with the computer letting you know how you are doing.

To the uninitiated, the readout (printout) from the machine may, depending on the way it is worded, give a false impression that this is an immediate personal message from another person, thus incorrectly and mystically "personalizing" the machine.

193 *Ouija* DD: 133.93 LC: BF 1585-1623 GV 1541-1561

The Ouija board has the letters of the alphabet, numbers, and "yes" and "no" printed on it. A wooden block which slides easily on the board is used by two players, each of whom rests his fingers on the block.

Questions are asked the board which answers according to the movement of the block in resting on the "yes" or "no" or in spelling out the words or indicating numbers.

Players are cautioned to be careful to try not to deliberately influence the direction which the block takes. Sooner or later movement of the block occurs. To the participants, the block seems to move itself because they are not aware of pushing it.

Sometimes very sophisticated and astonishing answers are reported by the board. Spiritualists tend to accept these as communications from people not present, either living or dead. Psychologists believe that the minds of the participants, without their conscious awareness, control the movement of the block through unrecognized pressures of finger, hand, and arm and spell out answers some of which (either consciously or unconsciously) are partially or fully known to the participant.

194 Real-Life Simulation Games DD: 658.124, 658.85 LC: 5549.T57-T58

Games which closely resemble real-life situations are used in managerial and training programs and in schools but are of sufficient interest to be pursued as an avocational activity. Players are given a set of conditions simulating situations to be found in existing organizations and decisions are to be made and solutions found. These have been used in simulating sales campaigns, and in teaching political science and many other subjects.

On a larger scale there are attempts to simulate a segment of the total society such as a city.

210 Professional Sports Observation

ENVIRONMENTAL FACTORS: indoor, outdoor, no specific environment, modicum of space, requires little or no equipment, equipment normally at hand.

SOCIAL-PSYCHOLOGICAL FACTORS: aesthetic, pre-patterned, concrete, individual effort, structured, unsupervised, little opportunity for recognition.

Impairment Limitations

blind	S1	balance	+	*hands impaired:*	*1*	*2*
low vision	S1	seizures	+	reaching	+	+
hearing	M2	*aphasia:*		handling	+	+
speech	+	receptive	M2	fingering	+	+
retardation	+	expressive	+	feeling	+	+
memory	+	mixed	M2	no hands	+	

impaired:

stooping	+	wheel chair	+	bed patient	+
kneeling	+	semi-ambulant	+	respiratory	+
crouching	+	Class III heart	+	*Energy Expenditure in*	
crawling	+	Class IV heart	+	*METS:* 1.5–3.2	

M2 may be able to see enough to understand and enjoy the event
S1   listening to radio or television

Viewing a sports event in person and viewing it on television bear few similarities. The two activities have only the sports event itself in common. Attending a professional sports event, the spectator enters a colorful environment of which the athletic contest is only a part.

The television spectator often has a view of the athletic event superior to that of his counterpart in the stands, but the telescopic lens of the TV camera cannot completely capture the excitement and richness of the sport being viewed, or of its live followers.

A visit to a professional sports event immerses one in the heady atmosphere which a large, loud crowd always creates. The spectator witnesses an intriguing variety of human behavior, dress and speech. Professional sport in all forms has always cloaked itself in an aura of glamor and drama, and if live spectators did not recognize this aura and seek to participate in it, professional sport would not survive.

There are some who believe that professional sports events constitute a ritual, secular but real, in which commonly held values are enacted in a stylized, larger than life scale. This is a moot point, but it is undeniable that a professional athletic contest, especially between rival teams, thoroughly captures the imagination of the live spectator and conquers his strongest social inhibitions. In the heat of a particular game, the normally placid, restrained personality can boil over into behavior which one might judge pathological in any other situation. To witness this phenomenon, or to experience it oneself, one must attend a sports event in person because no television image can suffice.

Each professional sport itself has its own delights to offer the spectator. In baseball, the slow pace of the game affords the viewer a perfect background for pleasant conversation. Attending a golf tournament is like a walk in a park or a large picnic. Football and large-scale indoor sports like hockey and basketball are the ones which lend themselves to the kind of hysteria mentioned above.

In any event, the experience of traveling to a sports arena and joining an enthusiastic crowd in its escape from petty cares is one which all ought to know.

The intellectual demand on the observer is that the person be aware of the rules by which the sport is played, i.e., knows how the winning score is attained, and as a supplementary activity, is able to read sports pages which contain reviews and summaries of the results.

A contest to predict scores established among the homebound handicapped who are limited to observation via TV or radio can be carried on by a telephone network which may get them acquainted and set up a framework for continuing contacts.

221 Bicycling, Motorcycling, Unicycling

ENVIRONMENTAL FACTORS: outdoor, no specific environment, unlimited space, equipment a major factor, equipment not necessarily at hand.

SOCIAL-PSYCHOLOGICAL FACTORS: aesthetic, creative, concrete, group effort, individual effort, unstructured, unsupervised, little opportunity for recognition.

Impairment Limitations

blind	0	balance	0	*hands impaired:*	*1*	*2*
low vision	S1	seizures	0	reaching	S2	0
hearing	M1	*aphasia:*		handling	S2	0
speech	+	receptive	+	fingering	S2	0
retardation	+	expressive	+	feeling	S2	0
memory	M1	mixed	+	no hands	0	

impaired:

stooping	S3	wheel chair	0	bed patient	0
kneeling	S3	semi-ambulant	0	respiratory	0
crouching	S3	Class III heart	0	*Energy Expenditure in*	
crawling	S3	Class IV heart	0	*METS:* 3—11	

M1 should have a companion along for safety
S1 protected area
S2 depends on type of hand controls
S3 may limit pedaling a bicycle unless under therapeutic prescription

221 *Bicycling* DD: 796.6 LC: GV 1041

There has been a renewed enthusiasm for bicycling for health and ecological reasons. Providing there are suitable roads or trails bicycles offer cheap efficient transportation and healthy exercise. Technological improvements have produced the 5 and 10 speed bikes multiplying the effectiveness of muscle power. Were proper routes provided, bicycles could be used for short distance inter city travel, substantially reducing the traffic jams and parking problems. A survey done in 1960 described it as ". . . almost altogether an activity of youth." "Nine percent of the population reported engaging (in bicycling) . . ." "Boys are more active cyclists than girls." "Nonwhites cycle more than whites." "Persons with limiting impairments cycle quite infrequently but those whose impairments are not limiting cycle almost as frequently as those who have no impairments."[9] For the year 1970 the State of Wisconsin reported 994 bicycles involved in accidents which resulted in 26 fatalities and 961 injuries.[10] Nation wide non-fatal injuries reached about 37,000 in 1967 of which three-quarters occurred to children aged 5-14.[11]

222 *Boating, Sailing, Canoeing*

ENVIRONMENTAL FACTORS: outdoor, specialized environment and/or climate, unlimited space, equipment a major factor, equipment not necessarily at hand.

[9]Outdoor Recreation Resources Review Commission, *National Recreation Survey*, ORRRC Study Report 19 (Washington, D.C., Govt. Printing Office, 1962), pp. 11-12.

[10]Division of Motor Vehicles, *Wisconsin Accident Facts 1970* (Madison, Wisconsin, 1971 ed.), p. 32.

[11]National Safety Council, *Safety Education Data Sheet No. 1*, rev. ed. (Chicago).

SOCIAL-PSYCHOLOGICAL FACTORS: aesthetic, creative, concrete, group effort, individual effort, unstructured, supervised, unsupervised, little opportunity for recognition.

Impairment Limitations

blind	M1	balance	M4	*hands impaired:*	*1*	*2*
low vision	M2	seizures	0	reaching	S1	0
hearing	+	*aphasia:*		handling	S1	0
speech	+	receptive	+	fingering	S1	0
retardation	+	expressive	+	feeling	+	+
memory	M3	mixed	+	no hands	0	

impaired:

stooping	S2	wheel chair	M4	bed patient	0
kneeling	+	semi-ambulant	M4	respiratory	+
crouching	S2	Class III heart	S3	*Energy Expenditure in*	
crawling	+	Class IV heart	0	*METS:* 1.6-4.0	

M1 could enjoy activities with companion to run the boat
M2 low speed
M3 should have companion along for safety
M4 should be seated and firmly restrained in position in cabin cruiser or pontoon boat
S1 power boat or as passenger
S2 depends on type and size of craft
S3 medium to large size power boat

222 *Sailing* DD: 797.1

There are so many eloquent descriptions of the joys of sailing that we will confine our few words to a more prosaic discussion. Like hiking, bicycling, and canoeing, sailing is ecologically desirable. Depending on wind power, it uses up no irreplaceable fossil fuel, proliferates no pollutants. Sailing craft range from small sailing "fish" which are essentially wood or canvas platforms on hulls or pontoons to ocean racing cruisers.

Although anyone can learn the basic elements in sailing in one afternoon, it is said that no one ever learns all there is to know about sailing.

The nature of sailing decisions requires a hierarchical relationship of authority between skipper and crew. When the skipper says "Duck! We're coming around," this is an order not to be disregarded. Among the experienced, the harshness is mediated by trading off as skipper and crew. Contrary to any land lubber's possible misimpressions, the crew has a lot to do and when things have to be done, they have to be done quickly.

A voyage in rough weather gives an exhilarating feeling of mastering the elements. Whether on land or sea, sailors become highly sensitive to the direction and force of the wind even during the course of their daily round of non-sailing duties.

222 *Canoeing* DD: 797.122 LC: GV 781-785

Canoeing offers an extremely wide range of possibilities from drifting around on a quiet pond to exciting and hazardous white water canoeing requiring substantial paddling power, skill and experience.

The shape of the canoe in which form follows function is an unending delight. The smaller aluminum canoes are very light and can be comfortably portaged. Canoes of all sizes up to guide canoes can be readily carried on tops of cars which gives them a wide mobility range without the turning and backing problems of boats hauled on trailers.

The canoe can traverse very narrow and shallow creeks and bayous inaccessible to larger crafts. These waters are often teeming with interesting wildlife and vegetation of all kinds.

In contrast to rowers, canoers have the advantage of looking to see what is ahead. Canoes can be paddled noiselessly so that wildlife may be approached more closely than in crafts which noisily announce their arrival. River canoeing includes the excitement of always wondering what is around the next bend: rapids? logs? rocks? bear? deer? turtles? muskrats? heron?

When river canoeing, it is more economical to travel in parties of at least two canoes because using two cars simplifies the arrangements: one car is parked downstream where the trip ends. For river canoeing it is essential to purchase a map, if one has been published, showing the canoeable parts of a river. Since poorly marked back roads are frequently the only means of driving to and from the river, it is well to mark and describe them on a map lest you forget where they were if you do the same trip next year.

222 *Rowing* LC: GV 791-809

Although many types of craft may be rowed in an emergency, rowing, as an avocational activity, is ordinarily done in a rowboat or scull in which the rower, sitting in the middle of the boat, propels the boat through the water by pressure on oars on each side of the craft.

The speed attained varies with the size and shape of the craft from sleek hulled scull to foul weather dory. Because of the leverage obtained, greater speeds are possible than in a canoe of similar weight, but the rower usually tires sooner. In rowing there is heavy use of back and leg muscles. The use of leg muscles is increased in a movable seat scull. The leverage obtained from oars inserted in the water about 4 to 6 feet from the boat and about 10 to 15 feet apart, makes for greater control and stability in high wind and waves than is available in a canoe. The position of the rower is awkward in that he faces backward and must occasionally look around to avoid other boats. The boat may be rowed in a straight line by sighting on two stationary points in a line to the rear of the boat.

224 *Horseback Riding* DD: 798.2 LC: SF 277-359

ENVIRONMENTAL FACTORS: outdoor, specialized environment and/or climate, unlimited space, equipment a major factor, equipment not necessarily at hand.

SOCIAL-PSYCHOLOGICAL FACTORS: aesthetic, pre-patterned, concrete, individual effort, unstructured, unsupervised, little opportunity for recognition.

Impairment Limitations

				hands impaired:	1	2
blind	M1	balance	0			
low vision	M1	seizures	0	reaching	+	+
hearing	+	*aphasia:*		handling	+	0
speech	+	receptive	+	fingering	+	0
retardation	+	expressive	+	feeling	+	0
memory	M2	mixed	+	no hands	0	

impaired:

stooping	+	wheel chair	0	bed patient	0
kneeling	+	semi-ambulant	0	respiratory	0
crouching	+	Class III heart	0	*Energy Expenditure in*	
crawling	+	Class IV heart	0	*METS:* 3.0-8.0	

M1 with a companion on the horse
M2 with a companion along

Horseback riding serves varied recreational purposes. Riding may be primarily a means to enjoy the scenery and the feeling of being out-of-doors alone or with friends. Owning a horse may be a vehicle for identifying with and belonging to certain "in" groups, such as the Masonic Horse Patrols, 4-H projects, or various riding and hunting clubs. Each membership is constituted of distinctly different social classes and occupational backgrounds. For some owners or riders, the training and care of the horse is the basic interest. Showing horses of any breed is an absorbing competitive enterprise.

Riding is relatively safe, provided that the neophyte receives basic instruction in controlling his mount, and observes a few safety rules around the barn and on the trail. Twelve weeks of once weekly competent instruction should be sufficient for most people who are only interested in occasional pleasure rides.

There are numerous light horse breeds, and breed associations are good sources of information concerning breed standards, lists of breeders, show circuits, and the care, training, and optimal use of each particular type of horse. Equestrian magazines usually contain many informative articles concerning proper riding techniques, show standards, and general information of interest to horsemen.

The dollar investment in horseback riding can range from a basic $2.00 per hour for the pleasure rider who rents a horse (this fee varies regionally) , to thousands in horses, equipment, entry fees and professional handling costs in the case of the wealthy dedicated amateur owner who invests in a "string" of show horses.

Physical requirements for riding are moderate. Although riding can be extremely strenuous, an individual can set his own pace and expend a small amount of energy if this is more desirable. Only a fair amount of motor coordination is needed for pleasure riding, but a rather high degree of complex coordination is required for riding five-gaited horses. Those with handicaps such as blindness, deafness, and loss of one arm have acquired sufficient skill to be able to show horses successfully. Balance is more important than strength when riding.

A rider should possess a fair amount of self-control and be able to have some sense of how an animal reacts to fearful objects. He should also know how his horse will react to different methods of control: the voice, reins, and the use of body weight and legs. He should be able to keep a cool head in such emergencies as may arise.

"A study of rural recreational accidents in Ohio found that accidents involving horses ranked third as the cause of injuries. Falls from horses accounted for more than two-thirds of the reported riding accidents."[12]

225 *Physical Fitness Sports* DD: 796.4 LC: GV 481, GV 341, GV 461, GV 511, GV 553, GV 1061

ENVIRONMENTAL FACTORS: indoor, outdoor, no specific environment, unlimited space, requires little or no equipment, equipment a major factor, equipment normally at hand.

SOCIAL-PSYCHOLOGICAL FACTORS: aesthetic, creative, concrete, individual effort, unstructured, unsupervised, opportunity for recognition, little opportunity for recognition.

Impairment Limitations

blind	M1	balance	0	*hands impaired:*	1	2
low vision	M1	seizures	S1	reaching	+	S1
hearing	+	*aphasia:*		handling	+	S1
speech	+	receptive	+	fingering	+	S1
retardation	+	expressive	+	feeling	+	S1
memory	+	mixed	+	no hands	S1	
impaired:						
stooping	S2	wheel chair	S3	bed patient	S4	
kneeling	S2	semi-ambulant	S3	respiratory	0	
crouching	S2	Class III heart	0	*Energy Expenditure in*		
crawling	S2	Class IV heart	0	*METS:* 3.2-22		

[12]National Safety Council, *Horseback Riding*, Safety Education Data Sheet No. 42, rev. ed.

M1 jogging and running in a protected area with a companion
S1 jogging, running
S2 some gymnatics, weightlifting at waist level and above
S3 weightlifting
S4 weightlifting for resistive exercises

With the exception of relay races and some gymnastics, these activities tend to be carried on individually, sometimes in the company of others. The object may be self-development, health maintenance or competition with others. The medical importance of exercise has become increasingly better known, particularly for middle-aged persons as a preventive against cardiovascular disorders.

Jogging is one of the simplest conditioning exercises available. It takes less time than walking. Because it is less strenuous than running it is better suited to younger people not yet fully conditioned for running and for older people. Jogging can be carried on almost anywhere, and no special equipment is required. Although there is a brief awkward period at the beginning when the jogger feels self-consciously that everyone is looking at him, eventually he learns to jog around town in business clothes when on errands without worrying what people will think.

Running takes less time but more space than jogging. It is probably the most efficient sport for young people to get in the maximum amount of exercise in the least time with the least equipment.

The term gymnastics is used generically to include setting up exercises, or calisthenics as well as the much more technically difficult gymnastic techniques themselves. Setting up exercises or calisthenics, like jogging, are primarily an activity for keeping in good physical condition and there are now specific guidelines by age and sex for scientifically selecting the proper exercises and the proper amount of exercises appropriate to each individual. Eventually the muscles get in tone so that exercise becomes a pleasurable sensation instead of an unpleasant series of aches and pains.

Gymnastics as a technical sport resembles tumbling, ballet, dancing, diving, and parachuting in the quite unique ways in which the body is manipulated through space. The body must be thought of more objectively and as more of an object outside of one's thought in order to control it in the complicated maneuvers it is required to make. Balance, timing and coordination all receive unusual emphasis.

Weight lifting is the muscle builder par excellence. It is time consuming, usually solitary, but more than almost any other activity, offers the possibility of the individual becoming a much more physically powerful person. Weight lifting is frequently pursued by boys, youths and men in search of an improved self-image, a more masculine concept of themselves and a striving for power through physical strength.

226 *Roller Skating* DD: 796.21 LC: GV 851

ENVIRONMENTAL FACTORS: indoor, outdoor, no specific environment, unlimited space, equipment a major factor, equipment not necessarily at hand.

SOCIAL-PSYCHOLOGICAL FACTORS: aesthetic, pre-patterned, concrete, group effort, individual effort, unstructured, unsupervised, little opportunity for recognition.

Impairment Limitations

blind	M1	balance	0	*hands impaired:* 1	2
low vision	M1	seizures	0	reaching +	M2
hearing	+	*aphasia:*		handling +	M2
speech	+	receptive	+	fingering +	M2
retardation	+	expressive	+	feeling +	+
memory	M1	mixed	+	no hands M2	

impaired:

stooping	0	wheel chair	0	bed patient	0
kneeling	0	semi-ambulant	0	respiratory	M3
crouching	0	Class III heart	0	*Energy Expenditure in*	
crawling	0	Class IV heart	0	*METS:* 5.83	

M1 in a protected area with a companion
M2 need companion to help put skates on and take them off
M3 slow pace

Roller skating is an activity pursued primarily by the young. Perhaps this is because they are more resilient, both physically and mentally, than older people seem to be. Younger people don't seem to worry so much about hurting themselves. Nor do they worry about looking silly if they fall. The self-consciousness that so inhibits older people doesn't yet affect them.

One's first attempts at roller skating can be quite frightening. The novice has to get used to moving on a set of four-wheeled feet, and until he does the ground or floor below seems fearfully hard and threatening. Once an equilibrium is achieved, roller skaters enjoy a new sense of movement, speed and balance. If finances allow, one can take advantage of indoor rinks and can roller skate all year round. Besides providing a controlled environment in which to improve one's skill, roller rinks set the scene for social interplay. The better skater can offer advice and encouragement to the hesitant. The fallen, victims of wayward and undisciplined leg movements, will be assisted to an upright position by helpful passersby.

Sidewalks are another of the skater's favorite haunts. Sidewalk skaters are a much more spontaneous (and/or much poorer) breed than the roller rink devotees. Sidewalk skating has one major advantage over skating in the rink; whereas the scenery in a rink is severely limited if not to say boringly repetitious, the sidewalk skater chooses his own view. The drawback of sidewalk skating is the greater safety hazards.

227 Water Sports

Water sports: e.g. swimming, skiing, diving, skin diving.

ENVIRONMENTAL FACTORS: indoor, outdoor, specialized environment and/or climate, unlimited space, little or no equipment, equipment a major factor, equipment not necessarily at hand.

SOCIAL-PSYCHOLOGICAL FACTORS: aesthetic, creative, concrete, group effort, individual effort, unstructured, supervised, unsupervised, opportunity for recognition, little opportunity for recognition.

Impairment Limitations

| blind | M1 | balance | M1 | *hands impaired:* | *1* | *2* |
| low vision | M1 | seizures | 0 | reaching | + | 0 |

hearing	+	*aphasia:*		handling	S1	S1
speech	+	receptive	+	fingering	S1	S1
retardation	+	expressive	+	feeling	S1	S1
memory	M1	mixed	+	no hands	0	

impaired:

stooping	S2	wheel chair	S2	bed patient	0
kneeling	S2	semi-ambulant	S2	respiratory	0
crouching	S2	Class III heart	0	*Energy Expenditure in*	
crawling	S2	Class IV heart	0	*METS:* 5.0-11.0	

M1 swimming in a protected area with a companion along for safety
S1 swimming, diving
S2 swimming

227 *Water Skiing* DD: 797.173 LC: GV 840.S5

Water skiing is unusual in that in order to ski at all the skier must first control the skis while the tow boat is pulling the skier to the surface of the water. This is an all or nothing situation where the skier either can or cannot do it. It can be socially embarrassing for those who fail many times because the failure is very obvious to all observers. Once up on the surface, it is relatively easy to stay up and to learn the more advanced techniques of steering the skis, riding over waves, etc., as well as the more difficult acts of riding one ski and jumping.

A 10 horsepower motor is needed as a minimum to pull a fully grown skier; a 25 horsepower is better. Spills may be dangerous at speeds greater than 40 miles per hour.

228 *Winter Sports*

Winter sports: e.g., skiing, sledding, tobogganing, snowshoeing.

ENVIRONMENTAL FACTORS: outdoor, specialized environment and/or climate, unlimited space, equipment a major factor, equipment not necessarily at hand.

SOCIAL-PSYCHOLOGICAL FACTORS: aesthetic, creative, concrete, group effort, individual effort, unstructured, unsupervised, little opportunity for recognition.

Impairment Limitations

blind	M1	balance	0	*hands impaired:*	*1*	*2*
low vision	M1	seizures	0	reaching	S1	S1
hearing	+	*aphasia:*		handling	S1	S1
speech	+	receptive	+	fingering	S1	S1
retardation	+	expressive	+	feeling	S1	S1
memory	+	mixed	+	no hands	S2	

impaired:

stooping	0	wheel chair	0	bed patient	0
kneeling	0	semi-ambulant	0	respiratory	0
crouching	0	Class III heart	0	*Energy Expenditure in*	
crawling	S3	Class IV heart	0	*METS:* 3.0-20.0	

M1 snowmobiling as riders; skating in protected areas
S1 skating, snowmobiling, snowshoeing, skiing
S2 skating and snowshoeing with assistance to attach shoes; snowmobiling as riders
S3 snowmobiling

228 *Skiing* DD: 796.93 LC: GV 854

The chief problems with skiing are the travel time required for most people to reach the hills with ski tows and the high cost of the use of tows. This decreases skiing's suitability for older individuals and other individuals with limited vigor who can only participate in vigorous activity for an hour or two.

The increase in the number of tows and the use of artificial snow are likely to increase participation in skiing. So will the four day week, locating more industries in the northern part of the country, and using school buildings year around so that more families will take winter vacations.

228 *Sledding and Tobogganing* DD: 796.95 LC: GV 855

With the increasing number of cars, fewer roads are safe for sledding. Neighborhood action is needed to encourage park commissions to plow park secondary roads and block them off to car traffic so they may be used for safe sledding. Few winter sports hold as much attraction for elementary school age children as sledding.

Tobogganing is one of the best winter sports offering family togetherness as a large toboggan holds the family. In contrast to sledding the toboggan travels successfully downhill and across fields. At best the steering capacity of a toboggan is far inferior to a sled or bobsled. The capacity to steer it depends on the amount of snow. On ice crust any effort to turn it from a straight course may well cause it to spin and spill all the riders.

228 *Snowshoeing* DD: 796.92 LC: GV 853

Together with cross country skiing, snowshoeing offers the maximum opportunity for wilderness travel without the noise and speed of the snowmobile. Used locally, every woodlot in winter offers the observer fascinating views of frost-covered bushes and trees. Tracks reveal the busy travel of commuting rabbits, and the intermittent tracks of pheasants. In our noisy civilization, few winter activities lead one so readily into areas of quiet and peace.

232 *Bowling, Lawn Bowling and Bocce*

ENVIRONMENTAL FACTORS: indoor, outdoor, no specific environment, modicum of space, equipment a major factor, equipment not necessarily at hand.

SOCIAL-PSYCHOLOGICAL FACTORS: aesthetic, pre-patterned, concrete, group effort, structured, supervised, opportunity for recognition.

Impairment Limitations

blind	0	balance	0	*hands impaired: 1*		2
low vision	0	seizures	+	reaching	+	0
hearing	+	*aphasia:*		handling	+	0
speech	+	receptive	+	fingering	+	0
retardation	+	expressive	+	feeling	+	0
memory	+	mixed	+	no hands	0	

impaired:					
stooping	0	wheel chair	+	bed patient	0
kneeling	+	semi-ambulant	0	respiratory	M1
crouching	0	Class III heart	M1	*Energy Expenditure in*	
crawling	+	Class IV heart	0	*METS:* 3-6	

M1 at slow pace

232 *Bocce* DD: 796.31 LC: GV 909

Bocce originated in Italy, allegedly a sport played by the Romans. It was brought to the U.S. in a refined form by the

Italians and here it has gained cross-cultural popularity. Many factors account for this popularity. The game is easy to learn, its trappings are kept simple—as long as there are eight balls and a place to roll them, you can play bocce. It's a game attractive to both men and women—in areas of high popularity there are community-sponsored leagues, just like the more universal bowling or baseball community leagues. There are different skills which come to play in bocce. Getting the ball positioned to your advantage may be done in one of four or five different ways. Devotees of the game have their own special style and playing the game gives them a chance to show their stuff. The game tests the skill of your own play and your ability to play against another's skill.

Perhaps the one feature of bocce which most accounts for its popularity is the atmosphere of the game. Unlike many competitive games, where silence is the rule of fair play, bocce players delight in the spirited taunts and badinage that are constantly exchanged during the game. Most often this is possible without causing hard feelings because the players are longtime friends. Devoted fans play bocce as much for the companionship as for the game itself. The love of bocce is so ingrained—most players are brought up with the game—that it is standard fare at picnics and most other family or social gatherings. Occasionally bottles of wine or penny stakes are added to the game to increase incentive.

233 *Golf* DD: 796.352 LC: GV 961-987

ENVIRONMENTAL FACTORS: outdoor, specialized environment and/or climate, unlimited space, equipment a major factor, equipment not necessarily at hand.

SOCIAL-PSYCHOLOGICAL FACTORS: aesthetic, pre-patterned, concrete, individual effort, group effort, structured, supervised, opportunity for recognition.

Impairment Limitations

blind	0	balance	0	*hands impaired:*	1	2
low vision	0	seizures	+	reaching	0	0
hearing	+	*aphasia:*		handling	0	0
speech	+	receptive	+	fingering	+	0
retardation	+	expressive	+	feeling	+	0
memory	+	mixed	+	no hands	0	

impaired:

stooping	0	wheel chair	0	bed patient	0
kneeling	+	semi-ambulant	0	respiratory	0
crouching	0	Class III heart	0	*Energy Expenditure in*	
crawling	+	Class IV heart	0	*METS:* 5	

The golfer is always playing first against himself. Getting the elusive birdie or eagle and lowering his handicap is the golfer's goal. But, due to the crowded conditions on most public courses, golfers seldom play alone, and competition is considered an intrinsic part of the game.

A great deal of coordination is required to play good golf. The beginning golfer is usually confused and frustrated when his instructor demands that he maintain the proper positions with his hands, arms, feet, legs, and body. It is, after all, the club that hits the ball! But the skilled golfer knows that every part of the body contributes to the smoothness and accuracy of the swing and hence the accuracy of the ball's flight.

Once the sport of the rich, golf is now available to almost anyone. Many municipalities maintain public courses on which one may play for a very slight fee; the disadvantage of these is that so many people have discovered the pleasure of golf that these courses are usually very crowded, and long waits are necessary before it is possible to tee off. That doesn't seem to bother the true afficionados; they rise at unholy hours in order to get to the course and secure a place in the waiting line.

The gentle exercise derived from walking around the golf course (carts, of course, provide an alternative for the non-athletic) is generally considered beneficial for almost anyone, and many golfers say that they are able to work out their aggressive tendencies on the frustrating little white ball.

241 *Badminton* DD: 796.345 LC: GV 1007

ENVIRONMENTAL FACTORS: indoor, outdoor, no specific environment, modicum of space, requires little or no equipment, equipment not necessarily at hand.

SOCIAL-PSYCHOLOGICAL FACTORS: aesthetic, pre-patterned, concrete, group effort, individual effort, structured, supervised, opportunity for recognition.

Impairment Limitations

blind	0	balance	0	hands impaired:	1	2
low vision	0	seizures	+	reaching	+	0
hearing	+	*aphasia:*		handling	+	0
speech	+	receptive	+	fingering	+	+
retardation	+	expressive	+	feeling	+	+
memory	M1	mixed	+	no hands	0	

impaired:

stooping	0	wheel chair	M2	bed patient	0
kneeling	+	semi-ambulant	0	respiratory	0
crouching	0	Class III heart	0	*Energy Expenditure in*
crawling	+	Class IV heart	0	*METS:* 5.83

M1 need companion to keep score
M2 use smaller court, companion to retrieve bird

Badminton is played by two or four on a small indoor or outdoor court. The players use small, light rackets to propel a bird, or shuttlecock (originally made by sticking feathers into a cork, now commonly made of plastic) back and forth over a high net. Because the equipment is portable it can be taken along to picnics and other outings if the participants are willing to dispense with a properly lined out court.

Although there are people who take their badminton very seriously, one of the nicer things about the game is that most people don't. Hitting the light bird back and forth is just so pleasant that many people don't want to interrupt the volley by scoring a point. The game is likely to become a cooperative effort to keep the bird aloft.

Badminton is a leisurely game, and conversation between the players is commonly both possible and convenient. Because the bird and rackets are so light, playing well requires a sensitive touch; height and long arms are also advantageous.

242 *Croquet* DD: 796.354 LC: GV 931

ENVIRONMENTAL FACTORS: indoor, outdoor, no specific environment, modicum of space, requires little or no equipment, equipment not necessarily at hand.

SOCIAL-PSYCHOLOGICAL FACTORS: aesthetic, pre-patterned, concrete, group effort, individual effort, structured, supervised, opportunity for recognition.

Impairment Limitations

blind	0	balance	0	*hands impaired:*	1	2
low vision	0	seizures	+	reaching	+	0
hearing	+	*aphasia:*		handling	+	0
speech	+	receptive	+	fingering	+	+
retardation	+	expressive	+	feeling	+	+
memory	+	mixed	+	no hands	0	

impaired:					
stooping	0	wheel chair	M1	bed patient	0
kneeling	+	semi-ambulant	M1	respiratory	+
crouching	+	Class III heart	+	*Energy Expenditure in*	
crawling	+	Class IV heart	0	*METS:* 3.0-4.0	

M1 possible but awkward

Croquet, a game that may be played by two individuals or two teams, has an aristocratic tradition. Thinking about croquet conjures up an image of a warm summer afternoon: young men in starched shirts and young ladies in long dresses playing languidly on a manicured lawn after a leisurely picnic.

In our more democratic era, the cost of a croquet set is within almost anyone's reach, and the playing field is likely to be someone's backyard. The game is played by striking a wooden ball with a short wooden mallet to propel it first through a series of hoops which are stuck into the ground according to a prescribed pattern, and finally to hit a small post with the ball. There are a number of competitive situations in which one player may strike another's ball with his own and drive it off course.

Croquet is a slow-moving game, the pace of which can be determined wholly by the participants' desire. It is not physically strenuous, and leaves plenty of time and energy for conversations between players. It would be especially suited to the individual who desires or requires some mild exercise but cannot exert himself too much; it is also easily adapted to suit various handicaps.

Avocational Activities

247 Tennis DD: 796.342 LC: GV 990-1005

ENVIRONMENTAL FACTORS: indoor, outdoor, no specific environment, modicum of space, requires little or no equipment, equipment not necessarily at hand.

SOCIAL-PSYCHOLOGICAL FACTORS: aesthetic, pre-patterned, concrete, group effort, individual effort, structured, supervised, opportunity for recognition.

Impairment Limitations

blind	0	balance	0	*hands impaired:*	1	2
low vision	0	seizures	+	reaching	M2	0
hearing	+	*aphasia:*		handling	M2	0
speech	+	receptive	+	fingering	M2	0
retardation	+	expressive	+	feeling	+	+
memory	M1	mixed	+	no hands	0	

impaired:

stooping	0	wheel chair	0	bed patient	0
kneeling	+	semi-ambulant	0	respiratory	0
crouching	0	Class III heart	0	*Energy Expenditure in*	
crawling	+	Class IV heart	0	*METS:* 7.1	

M1 need companion to keep score
M2 modify type of serving

Tennis is played by people of all ages and many social classes. It is a physically taxing sport, requiring a great deal of running after the ball, and provides good all-round exercise, but it *can* be played more lackadaisically, as is often done by players in late middle age.

Like golf, tennis is usually strictly segregated by social class; players usually play only with others of the same class. There is a considerable body of tradition and etiquette built around the game of tennis. The casual player may or may not choose to become involved in this, but he should at least familiarize himself with it in order to avoid committing faux pas.

There is tremendous psychological release in whamming the tennis ball as hard as possible, release found also in golf and baseball, but less frequently. Tennis is superior to badminton in this regard because of the heavier equipment. The "kill" in which the ball is slammed very hard into a section of the court from which the opponent cannot possibly return it is a legitimate way to release very aggressive and hostile feelings.

The scoring system used in tennis causes the tension resulting from the uncertainty about who is going to win to last over a longer period of time than it does in most games; once "in deuce" the game may hover for a long period of time over only one point.

Since tennis requires that a certain number of basic skills be acquired before the game can be played at all well, a few lessons from a professional or a talented amateur can be invaluable. Many municipal recreation departments provide tennis lessons at minimal cost.

256 *Wrestling* DD: 796.812 LC: GV 1195

ENVIRONMENTAL FACTORS: indoor, outdoor, no specific environment, modicum of space, requires little or no equipment, equipment not necessarily at hand.

SOCIAL-PSYCHOLOGICAL FACTORS: aesthetic, utilitarian, pre-patterned, concrete, individual effort, structured, supervised, opportunity for recognition.

Impairment Limitations

blind	M1	balance	0	*hands impaired:*	1	2
low vision	M1	seizures	0	reaching	0	0
hearing	+	*aphasia:*		handling	0	0
speech	+	receptive	+	fingering	0	0
retardation	+	expressive	+	feeling	0	0
memory	+	mixed	+	no hands	0	
impaired:						
stooping	0	wheel chair	0	bed patient	0	
kneeling	0	semi-ambulant	0	respiratory	0	
crouching	0	Class III heart	0	*Energy Expenditure in*		
crawling	0	Class IV heart	0	*METS:* 10-26		

M1 special rules

Wrestling, in contrast to most sports, uses nearly all the muscles in the body rather than a specialized set of muscles. Like running, effort for the most part is continuous and sustained rather than regularly intermittent like tennis or football.

Wrestling is an extreme test of the self. The participant is tested against his opponent within clear view of the audience. The outcome of the combat is entirely dependent upon his own sustained efforts. He cannot depend on fellow team mates as in team sports. An opponent's efforts may bring about sustained periods of discomfort and pain. If the opponent is stronger and more skillful, relief may be obtained only by giving up; consequently the degree of sheer perseverance that the participant possesses is more clearly revealed to the audience and to himself than in most sports.

Wrestling with no rules would be extremely dangerous and consequently a complex body of rules has been developed which are for the most part strictly adhered to by participants. Most of the rules must be carried out by the participants themselves because the difference between a legal grip and a dangerous illegal grip which may result in a dislocation or fracture may not be discernible to spectators and may be hidden temporarily from the referee. Loss of emotional control or psychopathic disregard for the opponent's safety can lead to disaster.

From the spectator's point of view, much of the time events move slowly, and because it does not attract large audiences, intrinsic rather than extrinsic satisfactions may be more important to the participants.

262 *Basketball* DD: 796.323 LC: GV 885-887

ENVIRONMENTAL FACTORS: indoor, outdoor, no specific environment, modicum of space, equipment a major factor, equipment not necessarily at hand.

SOCIAL-PSYCHOLOGICAL FACTORS: aesthetic, pre-patterned, concrete, group effort, structured, supervised, opportunity for recognition.

Impairment Limitations

blind	0	balance	0	*hands impaired:*	*1*	*2*
low vision	0	seizures	+	reaching	M2	0
hearing	+	*aphasia:*		handling	M2	0
speech	+	receptive	+	fingering	+	+
retardation	+	expressive	+	feeling	+	+
memory	M1	mixed	+	no hands	0	

impaired:

stooping	0	wheel chair	M3	bed patient	0
kneeling	+	semi-ambulant	0	respiratory	0
crouching	0	Class III heart	0	*Energy Expenditure in*
crawling	+	Class IV heart	0	*METS:* 14-26

M1 score should be continually posted on score board
M2 can play with one hand, although less effectively
M3 there are regular organized wheel chair basketball games

"Basketball has become numerically the most popular competitive team sport in the world. In the U.S. there are about three-quarters of a million high school players, including intra-murals."[13] It is statistically less hazardous than most other contact sports.

Basketball is a sport with a dual nature, depending upon the attitude of the participants. Basketball can be a mildly strenuous activity useful in integrating a small group and developing team-work; it can also be an extremely demanding sport requiring great stamina and development of special motor skills. Basketball can be a friendly game or a fiercely competitive one; the degree of seriousness of the participants makes the difference.

Basketball is a complex, highly regulated game. Few other sports limit the player so severely; basketball not only requires skills unnecessary to other games, but it also prohibits many movements natural to most competitive sports. In basketball the ball must be dribbled according to a highly developed set of rules; it can never be carried. Basketball prohibits physical contact between opposing players and requires a stoppage of play when such contact occurs. These are typical of the special athletic demands basketball makes on the participant.

Basketball, too, requires strategy when played properly. The sport has many elaborate theories, even a published body of knowledge, on tactics. Complex interaction between teammates is necessary for successful play.

The game offers a feeling of accomplishment, due both to the feeling of contributing to a team and to the opportunity afforded

---

[13]National Safety Council, *Safety in Sports: BASKETBALL,* Safety Education Data Sheet No. 77, rev. ed. (Chicago).

by the game for individual finesse. Few other sports have such frequent scoring as basketball; hence the game offers a high degree of positive reinforcement and reward for increased skills on the court.

Basketball need not be undertaken with such a spirit of competitiveness and seriousness. A basketball, hoop, and backboard by themselves, indoors or out, provide opportunity for varied athletic activity. A person by himself can practice shots and "moves" and one can challenge a partner to duplicate a certain shot. Such informal activity calls for less agility and less competitive motivation; as such it is well suited to those with minor disabilities.

264 Hockey

ENVIRONMENTAL FACTORS: indoor, outdoor, specialized environment and/or climate, modicum of space, equipment a major factor, equipment not necessarily at hand.

SOCIAL-PSYCHOLOGICAL FACTORS: aesthetic, pre-patterned, concrete, group effort, structured, supervised, opportunity for recognition.

Impairment Limitations

blind	0	balance	0	*hands impaired:*	*1*	*2*
low vision	0	seizures	0	reaching	M1	0
hearing	+	*aphasia:*		handling	M1	0
speech	+	receptive	+	fingering	+	+
retardation	+	expressive	+	feeling	+	+
memory	+	mixed	+	no hands	0	

impaired:					
stooping	0	wheel chair	0	bed patient	0
kneeling	0	semi-ambulant	0	respiratory	0
crouching	0	Class III heart	0	*Energy Expenditure in*	
crawling	+	Class IV heart	0	*METS:* 10.0-26.0	

M1 can handle stick with one hand, but less effectively

264 Field Hockey DD: 796.355 LC: GV 1017.H7

Field hockey is the only team sport played exclusively by women. It is one of the most aggressive women's sports, using much football-like jargon and emphasizing one-to-one defense. Yet, to be played well, it requires emotional and physical control by the players; field hockey is a game of precision movements, and fouls are called for even minor infractions of the rules. Field hockey is played in many schools and colleges, but in the U.S. it was introduced first in the Ivy League schools, and is still most frequently played at exclusive girls' schools. It is, consequently, a high-status game, although the equipment needed to play is not especially expensive.

Field hockey is usually played by two teams of 11, but can be played on a slightly smaller field with teams of six players. The size of the teams is one of the major drawbacks of field hockey as an avocational activity, since it takes 12 people to organize even an informal game. Additionally, playing positions are rather highly specialized, so one player cannot really be expected to learn to play more than one position well; it is therefore important that the same group play together regularly as a team. Field hockey combines the fun of an action sport with the "spirit" of a team working together to achieve a goal.

264 *Ice Hockey* DD: 796.967 LC: GV 847

Ice hockey, on both the professional and amateur levels, is primarily a man's game. It is a dangerous game, requiring strength and endurance.

Skillful ice skating is to ice hockey what running is to most other fast sports; no one should even consider playing ice hockey unless he is a proficient skater. The game is extremely fast and requires quick reactions; there are few breaks in the game, which is normally played in three twenty-minute periods. Ice hockey players are usually aggressive, and sometimes take their aggression out physically. Personal fouls are called, but these are small consolation for the player who has been hit with a hockey stick, accidentally or otherwise. Because there are usually no breaks between plays, there is no time for the players to cool down between incidents, and emotions often run hot and heavy.

274 *Foot Racing* DD: 796.426 LC: GV 1061-71

ENVIRONMENTAL FACTORS: outdoor, no specific environment, unlimited space, requires little or no equipment, equipment normally at hand.

SOCIAL-PSYCHOLOGICAL FACTORS: aesthetic, pre-patterned, concrete, individual effort, structured, supervised, opportunity for recognition.

Impairment Limitations

blind	0	balance	0	*hands impaired:*	*1*	*2*
low vision	+	seizures	+	reaching	+	+
hearing	+	*aphasia:*		handling	+	+
speech	+	receptive	+	fingering	+	+
retardation	+	expressive	+	feeling	+	+
memory	+	mixed	+	no hands	+	

impaired:

stooping	M1	wheel chair	0	bed patient	0
kneeling	M1	semi-ambulant	0	respiratory	0
crouching	M1	Class III heart	0	*Energy Expenditure in*	
crawling	M1	Class IV heart	0	*METS:* 15-26	

M1 if running is possible with any or all of these leg impairments

Foot racing may range from the informal spur of the moment races of children to marathon running. A recent report by Dr. Lawrence A. Golding of Kent State University in the May 8, 1972, issue of *Sports Illustrated* finds track competitors the most physically fit of all athletes.

The marathon distance is 26 miles, 385 yards, and the annual race in Boston is the most famous, with hundreds of starters. Marathons are run in various other parts of the country as well. In the midwest races are scheduled in Toledo and Upton, Wisconsin.

Long distance running is a unique combination of the mind (will) and body. The will to complete the task may give out before the physical resources of the legs and lungs. The will has to resist the impulse to give in to the combined stress of body aches, stiffening legs, blistering feet and burning lungs. The boredom of the long hours of practice required to build up endurance is an additional obstacle. Some anxiety results from the fact that performance is entirely up to the individual. There is no team or equipment which shares the responsibility.

Win or lose there is a tremendous feeling of accomplishment in going the route. It is the pleasure of having brought body and will to a level of maximum performance. A strong camaraderie exists among runners out of mutual respect for each one's efforts.

290 Miscellaneous Sports

ENVIRONMENTAL FACTORS: indoor, outdoor, specialized environment and/or climate, modicum of space, equipment a major factor, equipment not necessarily at hand.

SOCIAL-PSYCHOLOGICAL FACTORS: aesthetic, pre-patterned, concrete, group effort, individual effort, structured, supervised, opportunity for recognition.

Impairment Limitations

blind	0	balance	0	*hands impaired:*	1	2
hearing	S1	seizures	S2	reaching	0	0
low vision	0	*aphasia:*		handling	0	0
speech	+	receptive	S1	fingering	+	+
retardation	+	expressive	+	feeling	+	+
memory	+	mixed	S1	no hands	0	

impaired:					
stooping	0	wheel chair	0	bed patient	0
kneeling	+	semi-ambulant	0	respiratory	0
crouching	0	Class III heart	0	*Energy Expenditure in*	
crawling	+	Class IV heart	0	*METS:* 3-15	

S1 could do curling and soap box derby
S2 could do curling

292 Roller Derby DD: 796.21 LC: GV 851

The actual participants in Roller Derby are better actors than skaters; there is no pretense of art in either role. However, of more interest to us than the skaters are the spectators, in particular, the home fans who absorb themselves weekly in the roller derby spectacle. It is hard to define the audience, but one might hazard a guess that many are not sports fans. They disdain the American phenomenon of avid TV sports watching. They appreciate "Roller Derby" as a parody of TV sports with all its pomp and ritual. Roller Derby enjoys its own ludicrous rituals and displays. It seems hard to imagine that anyone takes it seriously. In this respect it is not unlike Big Time Wrestling. One suspects they share the same audience.

310 Passive Enjoyment of Scenery and Wildlife DD: 719 LC: BH 301.N3

ENVIRONMENTAL FACTORS: indoor, outdoor, no specific environment, modicum of space, requires little or no equipment, equipment normally at hand.

SOCIAL-PSYCHOLOGICAL FACTORS: aesthetic, pre-patterned, concrete, individual effort, unstructured, unsupervised, little opportunity for recognition.

Impairment Limitations

blind	S1	balance	+	*hands impaired:*	1	2
low vision	S1	seizures	+	reaching	+	+
hearing	+	*aphasia:*		handling	+	+
speech	+	receptive	+	fingering	+	+
retardation	+	expressive	+	feeling	+	+
memory	+	mixed	+	no hands	+	

impaired:

stooping	+	wheel chair	+	bed patient	M1
kneeling	+	semi-ambulant	+	respiratory	+
crouching	+	Class III heart	+	*Energy Expenditure in*	
crawling	+	Class IV heart	+	*METS:* 1.6-3.2	

S1   can hear, smell and feel some of the stimuli
M1   may be wheeled to view from a window or onto a porch

Anyone unable to appreciate the beauties and wonders of the world around him would be deprived of what is probably the most universal aesthetic pleasure, the enjoyment of scenery and wildlife. It is important that the severely handicapped person become aware that there is great pleasure to be derived from the passive enjoyment of scenery and wildlife. The inability to go for a solitary walk in the woods does not preclude the enjoyment of the natural world.

Scenery and wildlife can be observed throughout the year from within the home. Birds and small local animals can be attracted if food is put out for them; in time some will become quite tame as they learn that they will be safe with and around certain people. The interested individual can learn to identify various types of birds and animals and to anticipate the visits of migratory birds. Observation generates wonder at the nature of plant growth and change.

Much of the same natural wildlife observed from the window can be observed from a stationary position outside the home. A wider range of scenery will probably be observable, including such things as cloud formations. Being outside will also bring increased awareness and appreciation of climactic changes—warm sun, cool breezes, the stillness of the air or the quality of the atmosphere before a storm.

When removed from the home setting to a park or cottage, the individual has an opportunity to observe new types of natural life, and of course, new scenery. The careful observer will be able to note developmental stages which are simultaneous with or different from those of his home territory, while he acquires new ideas about the general nature of plants and animals. Traveling provides similar opportunities for observation and comparison, while adding the pleasurable sense of getting a more widespread view of the natural world.

Once the enthusiasm for the observation of scenery and wildlife has been aroused the individual has many resources around him for vicarious enjoyment and for learning more about what he has observed. Television and radio documentaries and travelogues, books, films, and records, lectures, movies and demonstrations can all add to his knowledge and to his thirst for more knowledge about the natural world.

The passive enjoyment of scenery and wildlife is primarily an individual occupation with little opportunity for social interaction. It can be a shared activity, and the severely handicapped person may require some assistance, but it is primarily a solitary pastime. Its chief value would be for the individual whose activity is severely limited and who needs an interest outside himself.

320 Observation, Exploration or Discovery Activities DD: 796.5

ENVIRONMENTAL FACTORS: outdoor, specialized environment and/or climate, unlimited space, requires little or no equipment, equipment normally at hand.

SOCIAL-PSYCHOLOGICAL FACTORS: aesthetic, pre-patterned, concrete, group effort, individual effort, unstructured, unsupervised, little opportunity for recognition.

Impairment Limitations

blind	M1	balance	S1	*hands impaired:*	1	2
low vision	M2	seizures	S1	reaching	+	+
hearing	M3	*aphasia:*		handling	+	+
speech	+	receptive	+	fingering	+	+
retardation	+	expressive	+	feeling	+	S4
memory	M4	mixed	+	no hands	+	

impaired:					
stooping	S2	wheel chair	S3	bed patient	0
kneeling	S2	semi-ambulant	S3	respiratory	S3
crouching	S2	Class III heart	S3	*Energy Expenditure in*	
crawling	S2	Class IV heart	0	*METS:* 1.5-9.0	

M1 would enjoy walking, hearing, smelling, feeling with a companion-guide, at slow pace

M2 could enjoy observation of large objects; avoid dangerous areas requiring good vision

M3 avoid areas where alertness to sound is important for safety

M4 need companion to avoid getting lost

S1 need companion for safety

S2 all but caves and other dangerous terrain

S3 smooth surfaced level walks

S4 avoid sharp rocks, etc.

The appeal of these activities would be more obvious to those who find a joyful fascination in the variety and splendor of objects in their natural state. The day's "find" might be rocks, shells, wood pieces, or a prolonged study of tiny clams burying themselves at the seaside. Equipment is minimal—containers for the compulsive collector, otherwise just one's eyes and a certain receptiveness. The affinity for this type of activity is usually ingrained, but at times acquired from the example of some other devotee of this quiet repast. As this quiet appreciation is a quality that can be developed, and grows greater when shared, the opportunities for creating bonds quite readily present themselves.

These activities call for no strenuous exertion, no specially developed coordination or muscle skills. The physical demands made are those of walking at whatever pace desired, bending over, picking up relatively light objects. While even these are beyond the capabilities of the bedridden, they are not impossible for the wheelchair patient. With minor adjustments, and an agreeable companion, the only somewhat physically disabled can explore, discover, and collect whatever type of outdoor inhabitant, animate or inanimate, most strikes his fancy. Certainly, unless one experiences a total aversion to the elements, the physical trappings of this outdoor lab should be not only pleasant but healthful.

The range of physical settings caters to a variety of personal perferences and available environments. Some require proximity to very particular settings; with most others finding the proper environment shouldn't be too difficult.

The activity may be goal-oriented—to find a particular stone or tree, to observe a particular bird, or may thrive on its lack of direction. The activity may be exercised within a structured group (a wide game or a guided nature hike) or at the whim of the individual.

For some the activity goes beyond the realm of avocation and becomes a profession in earnest. Or the activity remains avocational, but is reinforced by research and further education on the subject—the Audubon Society, identification and cataloguing of shells, rocks and semi-precious stones. Even at this level of increased concentration the demands made do not require great physical, intellectual, or technical abilities.

One danger of which the explorer must be aware is poisonous plants. "There are more than 60 varieties of plants in the United States which may cause irritation to the skin. Most persons are immune to the effects of the majority of those plants, but nearly every person who touches poison ivy, poison oak, or poison sumac is affected to some degree."[14]

340 Camping

ENVIRONMENTAL FACTORS: outdoor, specialized environment and/or climate, unlimited space, equipment a major factor, equipment not necessarily at hand.

---

[14]National Safety Council, *Poisonous Plants,* Safety Education Data Sheet No. 8, rev. ed. (Chicago, National Safety Council, 1946).

SOCIAL-PSYCHOLOGICAL FACTORS: aesthetic, creative, pre-patterned, concrete, group effort, individual effort, unstructured, supervised, unsupervised, little opportunity for recognition.

Impairment Limitations

blind	M1	balance	+	*hands impaired:*	1	2
low vision	M1	seizures	+	reaching	+	M1
hearing	+	*aphasia:*		handling	+	M1
speech	+	receptive	M2	fingering	+	M1
retardation	M2	expressive	+	feeling	+	M1
memory	M2	mixed	M2	no hands	M1	

impaired:

stooping	M3	wheel chair	M3	bed patient	0
kneeling	M3	semi-ambulant	M4	respiratory	M4
crouching	M3	Class III heart	M4	*Energy Expenditure in*	
crawling	+	Class IV heart	0	*METS:* 1.6-4.4	

M1 companion to serve as guide and perform tasks necessary
M2 supervision for safety may be necessary
M3 special sleeping arrangements and toilet facilities needed
M4 at a slow pace with competent companions

344 *Camping at Public or Private Campsites*

Camping used to be an adventure in pioneering—a cooperation with the forces of nature as a means of survival. Now, however, on any given sweltering summer week-end, a man gathers rations, equipment, family and friends, packs them into an air-conditioned trailer, sporting more conveniences than one finds in the average household, and joins 50,000 other eager Americans in their pilgrimage to the wilds.

However tempting the urge to surround oneself in conveniences might be, the concept of camping is the ability to enjoy oneself in his natural surroundings with only the basic necessities. Properly supervised camping encourages imaginative inventiveness tempered with a proper amount of humor and a definite willingness to go without one's accustomed luxuries. This last factor is important from the standpoint that a person's adaptability to different environments will enable him to be at ease in any situation in which he may find himself.

As a group activity, an enjoyable camping trip depends upon

the cooperation among the campers to assure that everyone shares the tasks of setting up and maintaining a campsite. The small comforts gleaned from a community effort will be all the more appreciated because they are not taken for granted and because they are a tangible indication of teamwork.

The physical exertion of camping would perhaps prevent the seriously handicapped from participating because of extreme weather or outstandingly primitive conditions. Sleeping on the ground or limited bathroom facilities might be insurmountable difficulties for severely disabled patients, but for those with slight physical impairments, the average state park or commercial campsite would pose no great problem.

350 *Fishing, Trapping, etc. of Aquatic Animals* DD: 799, 639.2 LC: SH

ENVIRONMENTAL FACTORS: outdoor, specialized environment and/or climate, unlimited space, equipment a major factor, equipment not necessarily at hand.

SOCIAL-PSYCHOLOGICAL FACTORS: aesthetic, utilitarian, creative, concrete, individual effort, unstructured, unsupervised, opportunity for recognition.

Impairment Limitations

blind	S1	balance	S1	*hands impaired:*	1	2
low vision	S1	seizures	S2	reaching	+	M1
hearing	+	*aphasia:*		handling	+	0
speech	+	receptive	+	fingering	+	0
retardation	+	expressive	+	feeling	+	+
memory	+	mixed	+	no hands	0	

impaired:

stooping	S3	wheel chair	S1	bed patient	0
kneeling	S3	semi-ambulant	S1	respiratory	+
crouching	S3	Class III heart	S2	*Energy Expenditure in*	
crawling	S3	Class IV heart	0	*METS:* 1.6-6.6	

S1 dock, bridge, boat or shore fishing with a companion to bail and throw line and aid in catching fish; blind not required to have fishing license in Wisconsin

S2 dock, bridge, or shore fishing

S3 dock, bridge, shore or boating fishing; ice fishing once the hole is broken

M1 with assistance of companion for throwing line

Fishing, with the exception of electronic gear for locating shoals of fish, has remained, delightfully, an art rather than a science. One of its charms is the large element of chance or luck which equalizes somewhat the success outcome of the experienced fisherman vs. the novice. That the drama takes place under water and in most cases out of sight adds to the mystery and suspense.

In fishing there is a vast amount of private lore to be learned upon which the fisherman does not have to submit to being tested on objective examinations. He may have the satisfaction of believing that no one else knows as much as he about the terrain at the bottom of his favorite fishing cove and the habits of the fish who dwell there. This is one activity in our culture where the individual is free to be irrational, emotional and unevaluated in his knowledge.

It may be argued that the American work ethic surrounds with suspicion and twinges of guilt anyone caught doing nothing. It is possible that fishing, which overtly appears as doing something, covertly permits the individual to do nothing, as he desires, and still appear respectable to himself and others.

"Preference for fishing (54%) is highest in the 25 to 44 age group. This is true for males, but females in each age group (to 65 and over) prefer swimming and picnicking to fishing."[15] "As a general practice males prefer fishing (47%) even over swimming (40%). Females prefer swimming (43%), driving for pleasure (31%), and sightseeing (24%) as well as picnicking (47%) in preference to fishing (21%) ."[15]

The sense of touch is highly developed in fishing and the experienced fisherman develops a keen sense of what's going on at the bottom of the water through the feel of the line. To the sensitive, this opens up a whole new world. He suddenly appreciates the scope of the many things happening under water obscured from usual human observation. The fisherman, through the feel of the line, is partially admitted to an understanding of these happenings. Fishing is a very cruel sport from the standpoint of the

---

[15]Outdoor Recreation Resources Review Commission, *National Recreation Survey*, ORRRC Study Report 19 (Washington, D.C., Gov't Printing Office, 1962) , p. 29.

fish and the bait. Most fishermen are able to compartmentalize this by assuming that fish and bait have such a primitive neurological system that they feel no pain. For the fisherman, protection against rain, cold, sun and insects is advisable. Finally, don't forget to get a fishing license!

370 *Raising, Caring For and Breeding of Plants* DD: 635 LC: SB

ENVIRONMENTAL FACTORS: indoor, outdoor, specialized environment and/or climate, modicum of space, unlimited space, requires little or no equipment, equipment a major factor, equipment normally at hand, equipment not necessarily at hand.

SOCIAL-PSYCHOLOGICAL FACTORS: aesthetic, utilitarian, creative, concrete, individual effort, unstructured, unsupervised, opportunity for recognition, little opportunity for recognition.

Impairment Limitations

blind	M1, S1	balance	S2	*hands impaired:*	1	2
low vision	M1	seizures	M1	reaching	+	S3
hearing	+	*aphasia:*		handling	+	0
speech	+	receptive	+	fingering	+	0
retardation	+	expressive	+	feeling	+	+
memory	+	mixed	+	no hands	0	

impaired:					
stooping	S2	wheel chair	S2	bed patient	S3
kneeling	S2	semi-ambulant	S2	respiratory	M2
crouching	S2	Class III heart	+	*Energy Expenditure in*	
crawling	S2	Class IV heart	0	*METS:* 2-8	

M1 avoid some power equipment like cultivators and power lawn mowers
M2 must be careful of pollen and irritating pesticides
S1 except mowing lawns and related yard work
S2 those which can be done seated, such as raising and caring for house plants, breeding and grafting activities
S3 raising and caring for house plants, breeding and grafting activities

Gardening is an avocational activity which can be carried on at many different levels of complexity and which can be adjusted to suit the needs and abilities of the individual. Whether he limits himself to a few potted plants on a windowsill or extends his activities to the cultivation of a wide variety of fruits and vegetables, almost anyone can develop a green thumb and experience the peculiarly human delight which man takes in nurturing growing things.

Although gardening is in many ways a solitary activity, it does have social aspects. The enthusiast will find garden clubs in almost any community; these can serve as a forum for the exchange of ideas as well as cuttings and slips. Plant care can be a satisfying shared activity; people working together with the same goal and caring for and about the same plant cannot help coming to care about each other as well.

For the individual who tends to be anxious or nervous, gardening can be a particularly soothing activity, bringing its own kind of peace. Plants, so dependent upon the natural seasonal cycle, can rarely be hurried, and the gardener will find himself working not against nature, but in harmony with it.

371 Raising and Caring for House Plants DD: 635.965 LC: SB 419

An indoor garden can be begun with a minimal outlay in terms of time, money, and expenditure of physical energy. Once enthusiasm is aroused, the indoor gardener can move on from simple, easy-to-care-for plants to the more delicate varieties, and will soon take pride in his ability to produce healthy plants and coax forth reticent flowers.

Caring for house plants is never physically strenuous: there is rarely need to fight the battles against weeds or insects in which the outdoor gardener must engage. The most necessary talent for this kind of gardening is the kind of patience which can watch a plant grow and develop and can take pleasure in the process without becoming bored or losing interest in the project.

The successful indoor gardener will soon discover that few gifts are more appreciated than a thriving young plant grown from an offshoot of one of his own favorites.

380 Animal Care, Training, Breeding and Exhibiting DD: 636.638 LC: SF 263-269, SF 106-121

ENVIRONMENTAL FACTORS: indoor, outdoor, no specific environment, specialized environment and/or climate, modicum of space, unlimited space, equipment a major factor, equipment not necessarily at hand.

SOCIAL-PSYCHOLOGICAL FACTORS: aesthetic, utilitarian, creative, pre-patterned, concrete, group effort, individual effort, unstructured, unsupervised, opportunity for recognition, little opportunity for recognition.

Impairment Limitations

blind	M1	balance	M2	*hands impaired:*	1	2
low vision	+	seizures	M3	reaching	+	0
hearing	+	*aphasia:*		handling	+	0
speech	+	receptive	+	fingering	+	S1
retardation	+	expressive	+	feeling	+	S2
memory	+	mixed	+	no hands	0	

impaired:

stooping	M2	wheel chair	M2	bed patient	M1
kneeling	+	semi-ambulant	M2	respiratory	+
crouching	M2	Class III heart	+	*Energy Expenditure in*	
crawling	+	Class IV heart	M4	*METS:* 1.5-8.0	

M1 should enjoy and be able to handle simply having the pet around, and performing basic activities, such as combing, brushing dogs

M2 safe seating facilities; small, domesticated pets

M3 small, tame, easy to care for pets

M4 would enjoy just having the pet around

S1 small animals with small food containers would require fingering

S2 guard for biting, cuts from the scales, etc.

At some time in the life of the average American, the vestiges of Adam awakened and compelled him to tame and subjugate the lower creatures. This inner stirring produced the household pet phenomenon, starring a cast of thousands, the common goldfish to the mighty lion, depending on the wealth and eccentricity of Adam's successor. The more common fish, turtle, cat, dog, horse, and inoffensive rodent varieties comprise the vast majority of pets, although exotic strains of these species have at times been introduced by the more imaginative. These imaginative innovations have sometimes been extended to keeping poisonous snakes, tarantulas and jungle animals, as well as the less frightening but still extraordinary bears, deer and tropical birds.

Whatever the choice, caring for pets is not so casual a task as might seem from its extensive following. Most pets require special attention, especially young pets. While entrusting them to inexperienced human hands may not be so comfortable for the pet, the development of responsibility and concern for a fellow creature in the human is a desirable side effect. Most times the care required by the animal is not so specialized and difficult as to be handled by only a very few. The problem is mostly in disciplining the owner to attentive and proper handling of the animal in his care.

In many man-pet relationships, a strong bond of affection results. This occurs most often in the "boy and his dog" cases, where the genuine love and devotion of the two develops particular, lasting and admirable personality traits. The experience is not limited to dogs or boys. Many adults experience affectionate attachment to their pets, devote many hours in their care, take special pains in breeding them and showing them off. Again, the discipline required of the pet is equaled by that required of the trainer. One might say, then, that this taming and subjugating is reciprocal.

For those with difficulties in expressing themselves and their emotions, an openly affectionate, loyal and uncritical pet might start them on the way to developing human relationships. Even for the less socially inhibited, the demands of responsible, loving attention for a living creature strengthens socially desirable characteristics.

On another realm, those who are experienced and/or enjoy working with living things might turn to care, training, breeding of animals in its more professionally attentive capacities as necessary, demanding and productive work. While physical handicaps might be limiting factors, age, implying experience, might be quite an asset.

390 *Natural Science Activities* DD: 500 LC: Q

ENVIRONMENTAL FACTORS: indoor, outdoor, no specific environment, specialized environment and/or climate, modicum of space, unlimited space, requires little or no equipment, equipment a major factor, equipment normally at hand, equipment not necessarily at hand.

SOCIAL-PSYCHOLOGICAL FACTORS: aesthetic, utilitarian, creative, pre-patterned, abstract, concrete, group effort, individual effort, structured, unstructured, supervised, unsupervised, opportunity for recognition, little opportunity for recognition.

Impairment Limitations

blind	M1	balance	+	*hands impaired:*		1	2
low vision	M2	seizures	+	reaching		+	M4
hearing	M3	*aphasia:*		handling		+	M4
speech	+	receptive	0	fingering		+	M4
retardation	0	expressive	M3	feeling		+	+
memory	0	mixed	0	no hands	M4		

impaired:

stooping	S1	wheel chair	+	bed patient	S2
kneeling	S1	semi-ambulant	+	respiratory	M3
crouching	S1	Class III heart	M3	*Energy Expenditure in*	
crawling	S1	Class IV heart	S2	*METS:* 1.6-8.17	

M1 can read braille books, listen to tapes, records, TV and lectures
M2 can read large print publications
M3 can read books, watch TV demonstrations, go on field trips and do their own exploration, experimentation or observation
M4 can carry on inside activities by having special attachments to turn book pages, adjust microscope, etc. or a companion to assist
S1 can do everything but field trips for rock collecting and archaeological "digs"
S2 can do only sedentary activities

One of the strongest motivations of modern man is curiosity. When man's question "why" leads him to the observation and study of natural phenomena, he ends up in one of the natural sciences. "If it screams or howls, it's biology; if it stinks, it's chemistry; if it doesn't work, it's physics."

There are many books and magazines written at an introductory level which can serve to acquaint the avocational scientist with his chosen field. *Scientific American* is one magazine which deals with topics from various sciences at a reasonably sophisticated level but which only assumes a layman's background. The avocational scientist may graduate to the more complicated technical journals which are available at most college and large-city libraries. He may want to seek out lectures on topics which interest him and will probably find these abound in large cities and university towns.

Many of the introductory books contain simple experiments which the avocational scientist can use to convince himself of physical laws. He may also use these experiments to astound his friends, since they frequently appear to defy common sense.

Many people with scientific training in one area pick up a second science as an avocation. Relieved from the necessity of earning a living, the professional scientist may pick up a second science in order to enjoy it without the necessity of producing.

Although it is unlikely that the avocational scientist will make great contributions to any field, he does gain the satisfaction of an increased understanding of a natural phenomenon.

391 Archaeology DD: 913-919 LC: CC

Archaeology involves the study of past civilizations through the material remains of past human life and activities. Much can be learned about past peoples through careful study of their tools, art or weapons. Activities in archaeology may range from collecting arrowheads and other Indian artifacts found in your own back yard to the study of the ancient civilizations of Greece, Rome, Asia Minor, or South America.

Archaeology is probably the only field of all the natural sciences where the contributions of amateurs have equaled the contributions of professionals. Many of the greatest archaeological treasure troves were discovered by amateurs pursuing their hobby. However, much work and great amounts of patience are necessary for archaeological investigations. If the amateur should be lucky and discover what appears to be a major find, he should be cautioned to seek professional help. Much information can be lost by simply moving articles from their original positions, and much seemingly worthless material may be of major importance.

392 Astronomy and Meteorology DD: 520 LC: QB 801-999

Astronomers are known as "stargazers" simply because this is the major part of their field. Through the study of stars and other celestial bodies, astronomers hope to learn of the creation of the universe.

The amateur astronomer can be content with much more reasonable goals. Ever since the ancient Greek mariners grouped the stars into constellations, people have spent hours seeking to locate the pictures which the Greeks saw in the heavens. Since many of the visible constellations change with changing seasons there is a continuing change in the scenario.

Many of these constellations are visible to the naked eye if one knows where to look. With the purchase of a relatively inexpensive telescope, the amateur is exposed to many other wonders of the heavens such as the craters of the moon, the moons of Jupiter, or the binary stars systems. He can view satellites sent into orbit by the U.S. or study annual showers of meteors.

Many local societies offer shows at planetariums, large darkened rooms where the patterns of the heavens are projected onto rounded ceilings by strategically located lights. This frees the amateur astronomer from the largest inconvenience of his work . . . the fact that to view the heavens he must work at night.

Other problems to the amateur are caused by city lights which tend to render the fainter celestial objects invisible and by large buildings which obstruct views of the horizons. Thus a person living in a large city may be forced to travel to the outskirts if he wishes to gain an unobstructed view of the heavens.

Meteorology is the study of weather and the art of weather forecasting. Although anyone can obtain the U.S. Weather Bureau forecast by watching the evening news, it can be more fun to try to predict the weather without the news and then compare your forecast, the Weather Bureau's and what is actually the weather. Through the years many people have come up with widely varying formulas for predicting the weather. A radio station on the West Coast predicts the weather by counting the number of mountain goats on neighboring mountains. Large numbers of goats are taken as an indication of fair weather. Although this procedure may not be terribly scientific, its accuracy to date has been better than that of the weather bureaus.

For those with a more scientific bent, the library contains many books on cloud formations, barometric pressure changes and their relations to the weather. The amateur, after some study, could use these as aids to weather predicting.

393 Botany or Horticulture DD: 580 LC: QK

Botany is that branch of biology which deals with the study of plants. As an avocation, the field of botany holds much promise for anyone who would like to be the proud possessor of a green thumb. Flowers and decorative plants lend a colorful touch to any room. They can be used as centerpieces, conversation pieces or gifts for friends. Although plants require periodic care, the total time spent may be as large or as small as the individual wishes, simply by increasing the number and/or kinds of plants which he maintains. The beginner is probably well advised to start with some of the plant types which do not require very much attention and are reasonably sturdy, such as the ivies. A more advanced student may wish to concentrate on more delicate plants or plants which require special conditions of temperature, sunlight or humidity. He may wish to grow desert plants such as cactus or he may wish to grow tropical plants such as orchids.

The very advanced student may wish to breed his own strains of plants. This is done by controlling the fertilization and thus the eventual seed production. He may wish to grow a strain with a flower of a certain color and would do this by breeding plants nearest to this color with each other through several generations. Local or national flower clubs offer assistance to the beginner as well as encouragement in the form of prizes and recognition for those who create the best new flower.

Biological mutations in plants is an attempt to produce meaningful mutations in plants, increasing their productivity and the stamina of specific species. Research and experimentation with such mutations may have many useful implications in the ongoing effort to produce more food for the world's population. There are many factors which can cause genetic changes (mutations), including intense light, extreme cold, and radiation.

Biological mutation using radiation as the source requires finding a source of radiation and a qualified technician to operate the machine. In a hospital one might perhaps be able to obtain the aid of a physician.

There are two stages in the plant's life at which one may intervene with radiation: the seed stage and the plant stage (which extends from the moment and seedling germinates to its reproductive stage) . When trying to radiate seeds it is important to remember that the seed's shell may be impervious to soft sources of radiation like *alpha* rays, and that the experimenter has little control in aiming the radiation.

When seeds are radiated, the entire organism, not specific areas, is affected. This may be just what one desires, if one is trying to determine, for example, the effect of radiation on the growth of the whole plant, on its reproductive capacity, longevity, etc. On the other hand, in radiating a plant, one can radiate specific sections of the plant—flower, root, leaves or stalk or stem—and try to discover the effects of selective radiation.

Having decided upon the experiment, one should form a hypothesis as to the results one hopes to find; this will usually help keep the experimenter from straying too far from the experiment. The second step is to set up a meaningful procedure, allowing for control groups, as few varying factors as possible, and eliminating, as much as possible, sources of error. Upon completion of the experiment one should observe the results and determine whether or not the hypothesis was correct, and, if not, pose the question, "why?" From these results, it should be possible to devise another experiment to continue where the first left off.

If a source of radiation is not available, selective breeding is a satisfactory alternative. Desired traits can be bred in, and undesirable traits bred out. The basic information or background knowledge needed is not extensive; acquaintance with the studies of Gregor Mendel will give the individual a fairly good idea of how to begin. Patience is required of the individual who wishes to engage in selective breeding; success with a first attempt is rare.

395 *Conservation or Ecology* DD: 574.5 LC: QK 901-989

Within the past several years, many people have realized that, as a country, we are despoiling many of our most valuable natural resources. Pollution of air and water has become a matter of concern to many people. There has even been a change in that which is classified as "resources" with irreplaceable scenery now being added to the list. For these reasons, conservation and ecology have become areas of concern to many people.

Strictly speaking, conservation is an attitude which seeks the wisest use of natural resources; ecology is the science or study of organisms in relation to their environment. However, popularly, ecology has come to stand for an attitude of respect for the environment and an understanding of man's dependence on it. There are several levels at which the individual may wish to become involved. First of all, because there is a problem of public apathy on ecological issues, there is a need for people willing to work to call public attention to them. This can take the form of writing letters to officials, using voting powers wisely, and publicizing local conditions contrary to an ecological attitude. A second level of involvement may be an individual's efforts toward a recycling economy, since this is the direction in which we must move to protect our resources as much as possible, or towards beautifying the city, or towards wise use of resources. Many groups have been formed to foster this type of individual action, and perhaps the individual may be interested in joining one of these to make himself more effective.

On yet another level, the individual may wish to study the science of ecology. Given the current interest in ecology, the individual who has spent some time in study of the basic principles is frequently in demand as a resource person. Many people who are concerned, but do not know what to do about the problem, can be counseled by the person who has spent time studying the basic principles. Because of man's dependence on his environment, some knowledge of ecology is essential for any individual who in any way affects the environment. This includes all people who are living.

396 Geology DD: 550 LC: QE

Geology is the study of rocks, minerals, and the formations in which they occur. As a profession, it is used in predicting where to drill for oil or water, establishing solid foundations for buildings, and predicting mineral deposits. As an avocation its most frequent form is the collection of rocks, minerals and/or semiprecious stones.

The beginner is well advised to invest in a simple handbook

outlining the various types of stones and areas in which they are likely to be found. It is also wise to invest in some outdoor clothing and good hiking boots since collecting may involve walking considerable distances outdoors. As the collector becomes more advanced, he may wish to travel to areas where certain specimens are likely to be found.

Presentation of the collection is an important part of this avocation. Many collectors simply display their finds on tables or shelves, in the condition in which they were found. With the purchase of polishing equipment, the collector can take the rough stones and polish them to highlight their natural color and shape. In effect, the collector is now involved in the production of "gems." These "gems" can be displayed in racks or on shelves, or they can be used in the manufacture of jewelry or other decorations. Work of this type involves a good deal of patience and some manual dexterity. However, the collector who has the patience to persist has vastly increased the beauty of his original collection.

398 Zoology DD: 590 LC: QL

Zoology is that branch of biology which deals with animal life. It includes the study of birds (ornithology), the study of insects (entomology), and the study of fish (ichthyology) as well as mammals, amphibians and crustaceans.

Many people become interested in various areas of zoology through their observation of some particular type of animal. For example, a person observing a bird may become curious as to the various types of birds, their habits, and their habitats. He may be led by a study of feeding habits to the study of insects, or fish, or perhaps to botany.

Interests in this field may be as simple as collecting various specimens of butterflies from the neighborhood and framing them along with their specific information. It may become as complex as study of the migratory habits of bird species.

Zoology can also be explored by study at local zoos or museums where animals can be watched live or where evolution can be followed through the course of centuries in the course of an afternoon.

Libraries are a handy source of material, but the more specialized student may turn to societies such as the Audubon Society which deals exclusively with birds in order to find more specific information in the area of his interests.

410 Autograph, Photograph and Poster Collections DD: 779 LC: TR

ENVIRONMENTAL FACTORS: indoor, no specific environment, modicum of space, requires little or no equipment, equipment not necessarily at hand.

SOCIAL-PSYCHOLOGICAL FACTORS: aesthetic, pre-patterned, concrete, individual effort, unstructured, unsupervised, little opportunity for recognition.

Impairment Limitations

					hands impaired:	1	2
blind	0	balance	+		*hands impaired:*	*1*	*2*
low vision	+	seizures	+		reaching	+	+
hearing	+	*aphasia:*			handling	+	0
speech	+	receptive	+		fingering	+	0
retardation	+	expressive	+		feeling	+	+
memory	M1	mixed	+		no hands	0	

impaired:

stooping	+	wheel chair	+	bed patient	+	
kneeling	+	semi-ambulant	+	respiratory	+	
crouching	+	Class III heart	+	*Energy Expenditure in*		
crawling	+	Class IV heart	+	*METS:* 1.4		

M1 add more written information about the individual items as a memory refresher

Of all collection activities, the collecting of autographs, photographs, and/or posters is among the easiest and least expensive. Like any collector, the devotee of such memorabilia can decide how carefully to limit his collection, and what amounts of time and money he wishes to devote to it.

Autographs and photographs of family and friends can generally be had for the asking; much pleasure can be derived from mounting articles like these and tracking down family heirloom letters and pictures. The collector might strive to obtain complete sets or a progression of pictures through the chronological periods.

Autographs and photographs of those in the public eye—especially entertainers and figures from sports or politics—can often be obtained by writing for them and enclosing a stamped, self-addressed envelope. Many people collect autographed personal letters.

Although autographed letters of famous people can sometimes be purchased (at prices determined by demand and supply), it is challenging to collect personal letters from public figures. This might be a particularly rewarding activity for the shut-in, bringing him a sense of connection with the outside world.

Although advertising posters can still sometimes be obtained free of charge, the great popularity of posters has turned them into big business. Most modern posters can be purchased at reasonable prices; antique and art posters are found in many different price ranges.

Costs involved in collecting autographs, photographs, and posters would not be prohibitive to any but the individual with the most severely limited funds. The only limitations on most collectors are time, and perhaps, available display area.

430 *Stamp Collections* DD: 769.56 LC: HE 6181-5, 6187-6230

ENVIRONMENTAL FACTORS: indoor, no specific environment, modicum of space, requires little or no equipment, equipment normally at hand.

SOCIAL-PSYCHOLOGICAL FACTORS: aesthetic, pre-patterned, concrete, individual effort, structured, unsupervised, little opportunity for recognition.

Impairment Limitations

blind	0	balance	+	*hands impaired:*	*1*	*2*
low vision	M1	seizures	+	reaching	+	+
hearing	+	*aphasia:*		handling	+	0
speech	+	receptive	+	fingering	+	0
retardation	+	expressive	+	feeling	+	+
memory	M2	mixed	+	no hands	0	
impaired:						
stooping	+	wheel chair	+	bed patient	+	
kneeling	+	semi-ambulant	+	respiratory	+	
crouching	+	Class III heart	+	*Energy Expenditure in*		
crawling	+	Class IV heart	+	*METS:* 1.5-2.5		

M1 possible with large magnifying glass
M2 add more written information about the individual items as a memory
   refresher

The pleasures of stamp collecting are varied enough to keep
the interest of both the devotee and the casual collector. Collecting stamps (or philately) surpasses many other avocational activities in two important areas: first, the hobby can be entered very
easily, with a minimum of expertise, intellectual ability, or
financial investment; second, stamp collecting provides opportunity for almost limitless involvement, with increasing personal rewards for more investment of time and effort. On any level of
interest, stamp collecting benefits the enthusiast educationally
and culturally.

The postage stamps of many countries are finely crafted minia-
ture works of art. The aesthetic value alone of many of these
stamps makes them worth collecting (interestingly, the United
States has never been noted for the beauty of its postage stamps).
Stamps, too, are extremely instructive of the history, customs, folklore, and economic systems of the countries of the world. Thus the
philatelist is led to an increased knowledge of the world and its
many cultures.

The key satisfaction of philately lies in acquiring a complete
set of the stamps of certain countries, denominations, or historical
periods. This is a goal seldom reached by more than a few collectors, due to the high cost and rarity of certain stamps. But the
nagging vacant spaces in the collector's catalog keep him searching
for the stamps he needs, even if complete success is unattainable.

Almost all acquisition of stamps is done by mail through stamp
distributors. These distributors send stamps to collectors on an
"approval" basis whereby the collector pays for stamps he wishes
to keep and returns the rest. The more stamps a customer-collector
buys, the more varied and valuable stamps the distributor sends
him. Hence, this "approval" system constantly renews the interest
of the collector, allowing him to pursue his hobby to any level he
desires. Continued interest in stamps necessitates increasingly
more expensive stamps.

Philately is largely a solitary activity, offering little opportunity for direct social interaction. Thousands of stamp clubs in the United States, however, do provide a social outlet for collectors. A wide variety of philatelic publications can give sedentary, home-bound collectors some link with the outside world.

The stamp collector is not often boastful of his hobby because of general indifference to it. Typically, the avid collector keeps his enthusiasm to himself rather than trying to share it with a public whose lack of appreciation he cannot understand.

440 Natural Objects Collections DD: 579 LC: QL 63

ENVIRONMENTAL FACTORS: outdoor, specialized environment and/or climate, unlimited space, requires little or no equipment, equipment normally at hand.

SOCIAL-PSYCHOLOGICAL FACTORS: aesthetic, creative, concrete, individual effort, unstructured, unsupervised, opportunity for recognition.

Impairment Limitations

blind	0	balance	+	*hands impaired:*	1	2
low vision	0	seizures	+	reaching	+	0
hearing	+	*aphasia:*		handling	+	0
speech	+	receptive	+	fingering	+	0
retardation	+	expressive	+	feeling	+	+
memory	M1	mixed	+	no hands	0	

impaired:

stooping	S1	wheel chair	0	bed patient	0
kneeling	S1	semi-ambulant	0	respiratory	M2
crouching	S1	Class III heart	M2	*Energy Expenditure in*	
crawling	+	Class IV heart	0	*METS:* 1.4-4.5	

M1 add more written information about the individual items as a memory refresher
M2 at slow pace on easy terrain
Ratings assume making field trips to collect the objects; if objects are collected by others and merely classified and mounted at home, then ratings will be similar to those for 410, 420 and 430.
S1 collection of leaves, needles, etc., no running

With all collection there exists an unwritten but nonetheless compelling stipulation that the would-be collector be somewhat compulsive. It may well be that interest in collections is as much due to the drive sheerly to acquire and complete a collection as it is due to interest in the object collected. With natural objects collections, the interest in nature and the natural can be incentive enough.

Collections lend themselves equally well to the amateur and the professional and all gradations in between. While the aim of this inventory is to offer suggestions for avocational activities, and therefore, one might think that mention of a professional capacity is superfluous, still there is a purpose served in mentioning the more specialized or technical aspects of an activity—if only to remind one of the scope and diversity of any project and to keep one open to the many possibilities of adaptations and variations within an activity. This caution not to limit serves its purpose in considering avocational activities. In reference to this range of purpose and ability within an activity, butterfly collecting, an activity of apparently simple proportions, becomes, when carried to an extreme, a very specialized and informed study of butterflies: their migratory habits, structure, transformation, etc.

450 *Model Collections* DD: 623-629, 738-739 LC: NK 492

ENVIRONMENTAL FACTORS: indoor, no specific environment, modicum of space, equipment a major factor, equipment not necessarily at hand.

SOCIAL-PSYCHOLOGICAL FACTORS: aesthetic, pre-patterned, concrete, group effort, individual effort, structured, unsupervised, opportunity for recognition.

Impairment Limitations

blind	0	balance	+	*hands impaired:*	*1*	*2*
low vision	+	seizures	+	reaching	+	+
hearing	+	*aphasia:*		handling	+	0
speech	+	receptive	+	fingering	+	0
retardation	+	expressive	+	feeling	+	M2
memory	M1	mixed	+	no hands	0	

impaired:					
stooping	+	wheel chair	+	bed patient	+
kneeling	+	semi-ambulant	+	respiratory	+
crouching	+	Class III heart	+	*Energy Expenditure in*	
crawling	+	Class IV heart	+	*METS:* 1.5-2.4	

M1 add more written information about the individual items as a memory
  refresher
M2 avoid sharp objects

One who wishes to collect models is faced with the same problems of specialization which confront any collector. He cannot collect *all* models, and so must decide what particular type or types of models he will collect. He can first decide what general type of models he wishes to collect: model airplanes, animals, cars, ships, trains, weapons, or any of a number of other possibilities. Having reached this general classification, many collectors will want to specialize still further, concentrating on models of a particular type, from a particular time period or country, or fashioned from a particular material, e.g., English antique carved ivory dogs.

Whatever his decision, the model collector will find himself with ample specimens from which to choose. Shops which sell models are found in almost every community, and antique shops often have a selection of models and/or scaled-down toys which are old or for some reason unusual.

The individual with engineering or electronic skills or interests may become involved with working models of trains, planes, automobiles, etc.

Model collections lend themselves to attractive display, and the collector will usually want to show off his hobby and especially his latest acquisitions. The model collection can be quite inexpensive, or it can become quite expensive, depending on the sophistication and the desires of the collector.

Although not a social activity, model collecting, as a shared interest, can become the basis of friendships. Like any avocation, it does, at the very least, give the collector the confidence gained from achieving expertise in a particular area and so having some conversational material which is a little bit out of the ordinary.

460 *Doll Collections* DD: 745.592 LC: GN 455.779 NK 489

ENVIRONMENTAL FACTORS: indoor, no specific environment, modicum of space, equipment a major factor, equipment not necessarily at hand.

SOCIAL-PSYCHOLOGICAL FACTORS: aesthetic, pre-patterned, concrete, individual effort, structured, unsupervised, opportunity for recognition.

Impairment Limitations

blind	0	balance	+	*hands impaired:*	*1*	*2*	
low vision	+	seizures	+	reaching	+	+	
hearing	+	*aphasia:*		handling	+	+	
speech	+	receptive	+	fingering	+	+	
retardation	+	expressive	+	feeling	+	+	
memory	+	mixed	+	no hands	0		

impaired:

stooping	+	wheel chair	+	bed patient	+
kneeling	+	semi-ambulant	+	respiratory	+
crouching	+	Class III heart	+	*Energy Expenditure in*	
crawling	+	Class IV heart	+	*METS:* 1.5-2.4	

Dolls are certainly the most universal of all manufactured toys. In nearly every human culture, children play with models of the human form. In many cultures, dolls take on far deeper meanings; in our own, the difference between toys and symbolic images of religious and political significance is the difference between dolls and statues. Whatever their significance, dolls are always some kind of an expression of the culture in which they are made and used.

Many people of both sexes are fascinated by dolls and collect them. There is a delightful variety of dolls available, often at low cost.

Because of the aesthetically unappealing nature of so many of the toy dolls on the market (a parent has only to take an objective inventory of his daughter's playthings to become aware of their shiny plastic, vinyl-haired smiling ugliness), most collectors prefer to specialize in antique dolls or other specialty dolls. Fortunately, there are many of these available.

The collector who specializes in antique dolls may have been started on his collection by the discovery of a family heirloom doll or a doll which belonged to an elderly relative or friend. That's the way most collections of all kinds tend to start—with a discovery, gift or a single purchase. Having decided to collect dolls, a collector may decide to specialize in a particular kind of doll, e.g., dolls made from a particular material, by a particular process, or in a particular country. Very popular, too, is the international doll collection—collecting dolls dressed in national costume or in traditional bridal outfits from many countries.

Collecting dolls doesn't require any particular skill or ability or a great deal of money. Knowledge of dolls comes with familiarity. A severely handicapped person might need someone to do the legwork of hunting down new finds for him, but enjoyment of a doll collection doesn't require any mobility. The doll collector is bound to become interested in the culture which produced the dolls in which he is interested, and he will probably find himself looking into the history and techniques of doll making. He may even find himself making and/or costuming dolls, for his collection or for others.

Doll collecting, like many collection activities, is primarily a solitary activity. It would be an excellent activity for one whose mobility is severely limited. Since the objects dealt with are fairly large, doll collecting would be more suitable for someone with vision problems than, say, stamp or photograph collecting.

470 Art Objects Collections

ENVIRONMENTAL FACTORS: indoor, no specific environment, modicum of space, equipment a major factor, equipment not necessarily at hand.

SOCIAL-PSYCHOLOGICAL FACTORS: aesthetic, pre-patterned, abstract, concrete, individual effort, structured, unsupervised, opportunity for recognition.

Impairment Limitations

blind	S1	balance	+	*hands impaired:*	1	2
low vision	+	seizures	+	reaching	+	+
hearing	+	*aphasia:*		handling	+	M2
speech	+	receptive	+	fingering	+	M2
retardation	+	expressive	+	feeling	+	+
memory	M1	mixed	+	no hands	M2	
impaired:						
stooping	+	wheel chair	+	bed patient	+	
kneeling	+	semi-ambulant	+	respiratory	+	
crouching	+	Class III heart	+	*Energy Expenditure in*		
crawling	+	Class IV heart	+	*METS:* 1.4		

M1 add more written information about the individual items as a memory
    refresher
M2 need companion to move objects, play records, etc.
S1 china, glass, sculpture and records

Art objects collections appeal chiefly to the individual with a
highly developed aesthetic sense—the person to whom beautiful
things are important, and who delights in possessing them.

Taste is the single essential attribute of the art collector, but
taste can be, and frequently is, developed. While it is probably
true that nothing can replace childhood exposure to beauty as a
way of developing instinctive good taste, serious study of techniques, schools of criticism, and the historical development of art
forms can refine innate appreciation of beauty and, sometimes,
develop what was only a vague consciousness of beauty into a
keen aesthetic sense.

Different kinds of art objects appeal to different senses and so
to different individuals. Recordings—the music, poetry, and other
material that is recorded on them—appeal to the ear and the intellect; most other art forms are beautiful in their visual impact.
Recent developments in the production of record jackets—many
are now including drawings, unusual photography, poetry, etc.,
sometimes by name artists—mean that record collections may take
on some of the aspects of collecting visual art. The individual who
collects rare or beautiful books will probably develop a deeper attachment to those books which are by authors he respects or
simply likes than to those which he considers merely decorative
because of their bindings or illustrations. China, glass, and sculpture, all three-dimensional, cry out to be touched and felt; one of
the nicest things, therefore, about owning art objects of these
types is that the owner *can* handle them, whereas the museum-
goer can only look at them.

With all kinds of art object collections, one of the principal
difficulties is that they tend to be quite expensive. This is quite
understandable, in view of the simple laws of supply and demand,
but it is unfortunate nonetheless. Trying to build an art collection
with limited funds is always a frustrating experience. The individual on a very small budget had best limit himself to collect-

ing inexpensive pieces—folk art has a simple beauty of its own and can often be acquired cheaply. The individual with a sense of what is good in art is often able to purchase beautiful works from unknown artists for a fraction of the cost of a piece by an established creator—or reproductions. The latter alternative is not usually very satisfying, since reproductions, unless they are extremely well done are usually offensively crude when compared to the original. There are certain true art objects which are, in a sense, "mass produced," i.e., they are turned out by the artist in a fairly large quantity but of high quality. This category would include limited editions of books, prints, and etchings. Such art objects are less expensive than the one-of-a-kind variety, but the price will depend on their quality and on the caliber of the artist.

480 Antique Collections DD: 745.1

ENVIRONMENTAL FACTORS: indoor, outdoor, no specific environment, modicum of space, equipment a major factor, equipment not necessarily at hand.

SOCIAL-PSYCHOLOGICAL FACTORS: aesthetic, utilitarian, pre-patterned, abstract, concrete, individual effort, unstructured, unsupervised, opportunity for recognition.

Impairment Limitations

blind	S1	balance	+	*hands impaired:*	1	2
low vision	+	seizures	+	reaching	+	+
hearing	+	*aphasia:*		handling	+	M1
speech	+	receptive	+	fingering	+	M1
retardation	+	expressive	+	feeling	+	+
memory	+	mixed	+	no hands	M1	

impaired:

stooping	+	wheel chair	+	bed patient	+
kneeling	+	semi-ambulant	+	respiratory	+
crouching	+	Class III heart	+	*Energy Expenditure in*	
crawling	+	Class IV heart	+	*METS:* 1.4	

M1 need companion to move objects, turn pages in books
S1 dishes, glass and bottles, furniture

Fascination with the old is nothing new. Some people have always treasured heirlooms, either for their inherent aesthetic value or because of the memories connected with them. The popularity of antiques rises and falls, however. Some generations seem to be concerned only with the new; they are so taken up with the idea of progress that everything old is banished to the attic. But one generation's loss is the gain of the next, as children and grandchildren rediscover the beauty of the things that have been pushed aside.

Perhaps the popularity of antiques in the current era may be attributed to general feelings of insecurity brought about by rapid technological change which bring with them a sense of nostalgia and a desire to return to a simpler age.

Antique lovers are a special breed, sensitive to beauty and taking particular delight in the mellow loveliness of things which are both old and beautiful. The antique hunter must have a well-developed imagination for he must be able to envision his find as it will be when he has cleaned off years of grime and perhaps done some restoration and refinishing. He must be able to recognize basic structural worth and beauty of form in objects which to the uninitiated look like so much junk.

For legal and customs purposes, an antique is by definition something made before 1830, but in common usage, "antique" refers to anything old, outdated, or from a previous generation.

481 Books and Documents DD: 090.70 LC: Z987-997

Most antique books and documents could be considered as belonging to one of two broad categories: those which have inherent serious historical value and those whose value springs from their aesthetic desirability or from the fact that their original owner was in some way linked to the collector and which have historical value only insofar as they reflect the period from which they spring. Collections of the former type are of course more difficult to obtain and more costly, but even a single piece of this nature could be the pride of any collector.

Antique documents of a serious nature could include such things as correspondence between famous or important individuals, deeds, charters. Serious collections of antique books might include prized first editions, books which demonstrate new ways of using printing machinery, or even manuscripts. Other antique documents which might be collected would be letters between members of one's family, e.g., one's grandparents' love letters, family diplomas, deeds and certificates, old detailed account books, and quaint advertisements. The individual who loves books and considers them his friends will take pleasure in acquiring old books even if they have no great monetary value, because their makeup and content will give him an insight into an earlier age.

Unless one gets involved with re-binding, little can be done to restore damaged books or documents, so it is essential for full enjoyment that books be at least readable when they are purchased. The nature of documents will probably be known when they are acquired, but much of the pleasure of owning antique books is found in reading them.

510 Cooking and Food Crafts DD: 641.5-.8 LC: TX 645-840

Environmental factors: indoor, no specific environment, modicum of space, equipment a major factor, equipment normally at hand.

Social-psychological factors: aesthetic, utilitarian, creative, pre-patterned, concrete, group effort, individual effort, structured, unsupervised, opportunity for recognition.

Impairment Limitations

				hands impaired:	1	2
blind	M1	balance	M4			
low vision	M2	seizures	M4	reaching	M5	M6
hearing	+	*aphasia:*		handling	M6	M6
speech	+	receptive	S1	fingering	M6	M6
retardation	+	expressive	+	feeling	M4	M4
memory	M3	mixed	S1	no hands	M6	

impaired:					
stooping	M5	wheel chair	M5	bed patient	0
kneeling	M5	semi-ambulant	M5	respiratory	M7
crouching	M5	Class III heart	M7	*Energy Expenditure in*	
crawling	+	Class IV heart	0	*METS:* 2.9-3.3	

M1 use brailled oven knobs, braille cookbooks and taped recipes
M2 use large print cook books
M3 refer to cookbook more often, needs supervision, use timers

M4 protect against contact with hot stove, hot water, etc.
M5 store materials at waist level or above
M6 use reachers to hold things
M7 use appliances for prolonged beating and stirring activities
S1   can perform activities they already know, but can't read recipes or
     cookbooks

Eating is probably one of the oldest ways of socializing known to man. The idea of preparing and sharing food with one another is an accepted way of demonstrating friendship and trust.

Cooking, far from being unavoidable drudgery, can yield hours of happy creativity, given proper utensils and circumstances. Most people who hate to cook are those who are short on time and who therefore find getting a balanced meal on the table an arduous and thoroughly unpleasant task.

Since most people love a good meal, having the reputation of a top-notch cook is an excellent means of building self-confidence and receiving recognition. Cooking is also a good lesson in cause-effect relationships. You learn quickly that following a recipe and measuring proper amounts are essential ingredients in preparing any dish.

Cooking presents opportunities for group interaction. The preparatory stages of making a meal usually require an ample amount of chopping, paring, seasoning, measuring, mixing or grating, all of which are important and none of which takes any particular skill. As the cook gains confidence in his ability to prepare attractive, tasty meals, he can begin to create his own recipes.

Kitchen activity need not exclude anyone—physically handicapped, blind, or mentally retarded. Kitchens are easily adaptable to accommodate any of these, but special care must be taken with sharp or potentially dangerous instruments.

Some supervision would be necessary for a group of people to assure that directions are followed precisely and also to divide the various tasks. Cooking can be an excellent exercise in cooperation and team work and afford an opportunity for social interaction and create a common bond of successful achievement.

520 Decorating Activities DD: 642.8, 747 LC: NK

ENVIRONMENTAL FACTORS: indoor, no specific environment, modicum of space, equipment a major factor, equipment normally at hand.

SOCIAL-PSYCHOLOGICAL FACTORS: aesthetic, utilitarian, creative, concrete, individual effort, unstructured, unsupervised, opportunity for recognition.

Impairment Limitations

blind	0	balance	S1	*hands impaired:*	*1*	*2*
low vision	+	seizures	S1	reaching	M1	M2
hearing	+	*aphasia:*		handling	M2	0
speech	+	receptive	+	fingering	M2	0
retardation	+	expressive	+	feeling	+	+
memory	+	mixed	+	no hands	0	

impaired:					
stooping	+	wheel chair	M3	bed patient	M3
kneeling	+	semi-ambulant	M3	respiratory	+
crouching	+	Class III heart	+	*Energy Expenditure in*	
crawling	+	Class IV heart	M3	*METS:* 1.4-4.5	

M1 can do small objects on table or work bench and other things requiring one hand for reaching

M2 hold materials in vise, jig or fixture

M3 small objects on bench or bedstand

S1 all activities except climbing ladder to decorate Christmas Tree or install curtain rods

These activities are possible outlets for those who satisfy their creative urge through the medium of visual art. Certain concepts of artistic expression are crucial to this mode of decoration: a sense of form, color, proportion, composition. While some idea of the principles of artistic expression might be desirable or beneficial, they are not mandatory. Some people have an innate sense of the artistic and can manage quite well without formal instruction.

526 General Interior Decorating DD: 698.14, 747 LC: NK 1700-3505, TX 311-317

For most people, efforts at interior decoration translate into moving the furniture twice a year to add a little variety. For someone who has exhausted all possible combinations of furniture or wishes to delve more deeply into the possibilities of interior design, the requisite talents are more than the mere physical effort which suffices the biannual practicioners of the art. Basically, interior decoration is the planning, designing, and execution of an interior design. The explanation is more simple than the efforts that go into it. Good interior designing evaluates and uses to advantage the high or low points of the general structure. Consideration must be given to color and lighting, costs, materials, exterior setting, types of home. The decorator needs working knowledge of textiles, paints, wallpaper, paneling, furniture and flooring. An art major, or training at a technical or vocational school is a good start. Most of the projects may not be so extensive as to require all the skills listed above.

530 Interlacing and Interlocking Crafts DD: 746.41 LC: TS 910

ENVIRONMENTAL FACTORS: indoor, no specific environment, modicum of space, equipment a major factor, equipment not necessarily at hand.

SOCIAL-PSYCHOLOGICAL FACTORS: aesthetic, utilitarian, creative, pre-patterned, concrete, group effort, individual effort, structured, unsupervised, opportunity for recognition.

Impairment Limitations

blind	M1	balance	+	*hands impaired:*	1	2
low vision	+	seizures	+	reaching	S1	0
hearing	+	*aphasia:*		handling	M2	0
speech	+	receptive	+	fingering	M2	0
retardation	+	expressive	+	feeling	+	+
memory	+	mixed	+	no hands	0	

impaired:

stooping	+	wheel chair	+	bed patient	+
kneeling	+	semi-ambulant	+	respiratory	+
crouching	+	Class III heart	+	*Energy Expenditure in*	
crawling	+	Class IV heart	+	*METS:* 1.2-2.0	

M1 may need assistance of a sighted person
M2 may need jig or fixture to hold materials
S1 probably cannot reach rug frame

531 Basket Weaving and Wickerwork

The required skill is so easily developed that there are few who would have any severe difficulty in meeting the task. The usual material is raffia or wicker and the baskets, mats and assorted other containers that result from the shaping of these are both attractive and practical. If mistakes are made, they can easily be corrected. The materials are inexpensive and easily found. One might want to collect his own materials. Wood pieces and some sort of flexible yet sturdy reed are usually all that is required. Working on this level might encourage developing the skills in another field—weaving rugs, for example. One could allow for a certain progression of activity which would encourage the more capable.

532 Macrame or Knot Activities

Macrame or knot making activities: such as fly-tying or net making DD: 746.41. LC: TT 840.

The art of skillful knotting has come into its own with the sudden surge of macrame into the foreground of craft activity. There has long existed a close knot of skilled tiers who have spent their talents in the production of nets and, more notably, fly ties. For these, knot-making is no mere fad, but a highly developed art. The object of their intense craftsmanship is the simulation, as close as possible, of the particular bug, fly, or whatever thought most delicious by the fish of their choice. The more rugged may prefer its appeal to that of the more fashion-oriented macrame. Knot-making in any capacity can be the work of anyone, but probably the more patient and those given to appreciation of detailed work will first express an interest.

538 Weaving DD: 746.1 LC: TT 880-805, TS 1490-1500

Hand weaving requires a minimum of training and equipment. Simpler types of weaving do not even require a loom. When a loom is required, two weeks of instruction is considered ample time to grasp the technique. The benefits of the art are an interest in textiles and fabric construction, development of manual skill, and appreciation of textures and colors. Threading the loom is the most time-consuming part of weaving, but weaving is said to produce cloth faster than knitting or crocheting. Even on a small scale, metal looms turn out a surprising variety of items and are conducive to the exercise of creative design.

540 *Toy, Model and Kit Assembly* DD: 745.592 LC: NK 492, TT 154

ENVIRONMENTAL FACTORS: indoor, no specific environment, modicum of space, equipment a major factor, equipment not necessarily at hand.

SOCIAL-PSYCHOLOGICAL FACTORS: aesthetic, pre-patterned, concrete, individual effort, structured, unsupervised, opportunity for recognition.

Impairment Limitations

blind	S1	balance	+	*hands impaired:*	*1*	*2*
low vision	S2	seizures	+	reaching	+	+
hearing	+	*aphasia:*		handling	M1	0
speech	+	receptive	+	fingering	M1	0
retardation	+	expressive	+	feeling	+	+
memory	+	mixed	+	no hands	0	

impaired:

stooping	+	wheel chair	+	bed patient	+
kneeling	+	semi-ambulant	+	respiratory	+
crouching	+	Class III heart	+	*Energy Expenditure in*	
crawling	+	Class IV heart	+	*METS:* 1.2-1.9	

M1 if parts held in vise or clamp
S1 stuffed toy projects
S2 large pieces only

Toy, model, and kit assembly requires a high amount of discipline for success. As in every craft-oriented activity, model-making hobbies have ascending levels of skill from beginner to master. But almost all model making requires high degrees of patience, perfectionism, attention to detail, willingness to work systematically, and ability to know when and when not to follow directions.

Few model builders or toy assembly hobbyists consider these demands burdensome, however, because the creative fulfillment and recognition they derive from the activity reward well the meticulous care required by it.

Almost any kit assembly activity has enough built-in interest to inspire increasingly more difficult projects, mainly because of the hobbyist's pleasure in displaying his achievements. The more he and others admire his handiwork, the more he is tempted to outdo himself in his next effort, even to the point of improvising designs and personally surpassing commercially available model kits (This is where not following directions comes in. Sometimes originality demands diversion from the instruction sheet).

As the hobbyist gains more expertise in a particular kind of model building or toy assembly, he acquires a curiosity about the history and lore of his model specialty. In some cases, particularly among fanciers of model trains, this interest becomes almost obsessive, as the hobbyist seeks every available shred of information about his specialty. In his knowledge as well as his model making, the devotee considers no detail unimportant.

Model making does little to encourage social interaction. The activity itself is quite time consuming and requires extreme concentration; this is why model making and kit assembly can easily absorb energies which otherwise might be devoted to social involvement. Especially for those who have difficulty in social relationships, model building provides an excuse for seclusion. If the model builder or kit assembler receives deserved recognition for his efforts, however, his hobby can have positive social value.

543 Model House and Furniture Projects DD: 668.72 LC: TT 200

Model house and furniture projects lead one to curiosity about modes of living in different cultures and historical periods. Careful research as well as manual skill is required to enter this hobby activity. An eye for fine detail, too, is necessary if the model furniture collection is to have a look of authenticity.

544 Models of Trains, Cars, Boats, Airplanes, Etc. DD: 629.221 LC: TF 197, TL 237, VM 298

Models of trains, cars, boats, airplanes, etc. can be made in a variety of ways, ranging from commercially made kits to individually made-from-scratch varieties. In every case, the amount of the model builder's satisfaction is in direct proportion to his investment of time, effort, and expense on the project. Almost all commercially made models today are molded of plastic. For die-hard purists, model ships can still be purchased in wood, with fittings of brass and cast lead, but even the old salts must admit that plastic provides much better detail of parts than any other material. Beginners to the hobby should appreciate the ease of assembly of plastic model kits.

545 *Electronic Kits* DD: 745.59, 688.72 LC: TK 9971

Electronic kits enable the hobbyist to build everything from a toy telegraph ticker (suitable to late grade-school age levels) to the most sophisticated radio, stereophonic, and television equipment. A home craftsman can save hundreds of dollars in retail costs if he elects to make his own electronic equipment. Of course, the pride and satisfaction of one who makes his own stereo set are unbounded.

550 *Paper Crafts* DD: 745.54 LC: TT 870, LB 1542

ENVIRONMENTAL FACTORS: indoor, no specific environment, modicum of space, equipment a major factor, equipment normally at hand.

SOCIAL-PSYCHOLOGICAL FACTORS: aesthetic, utilitarian, creative, concrete, individual effort, unstructured, unsupervised, opportunity for recognition.

Impairment Limitations

blind	S1	balance	+	*hands impaired:*	*1*	*2*
low vision	+	seizures	+	reaching	M1	M1
hearing	+	*aphasia:*		handling	M2	M2
speech	+	receptive	+	fingering	M2	M2
retardation	+	expressive	+	feeling	+	+
memory	+	mixed	+	no hands	M2	
impaired:						
stooping	+	wheel chair	+	bed patient	+	
kneeling	+	semi-ambulant	+	respiratory	+	
crouching	+	Class III heart	+	*Energy Expenditure in*		
crawling	+	Class IV heart	+	*METS:* 1.4-2		

S1   working with paper mache is possible
M1   materials close at hand on table or work bench
M2   hold materials in vise, jig or fixture; may manipulate, painting, pasting
     implements held in mouth

A stack of old magazines, a sheaf of paper, and some glue and scissors can brighten the world of almost anyone regardless of disabilities or lack of skills. The whole variety of paper crafts can be be pursued quietly, at any pace suitable to the participant, with few considerations of financial outlay or space requirements. Even a small amount of imagination brought into play in paper crafts can produce delightful results, because most of these crafts are very simple in nature and seldom make heavy enough demands to overwhelm one's self-confidence.

Paper crafts, in their simplicity, play a highly important role in personal development: most children are introduced to the use of tools through paper and scissors. The satisfaction of using tools well is one which grows with most people into adulthood, of course. But there are those who "outgrow" the thrill of making things with hands and tools, or who have impairments prohibiting much handicraft work. It is for these kinds of people that paper crafts may serve as a vehicle of rediscovery. There is no adult who could not recapture, if he would only allow himself, the child's delight in using a scissors well.

560 Leather and Textile Crafts

ENVIRONMENTAL FACTORS: indoor, no specific environment, modicum of space, equipment a major factor, equipment not necessarily at hand.

SOCIAL-PSYCHOLOGICAL FACTORS: aesthetic, utilitarian, creative, pre-patterned, concrete, individual effort, unstructured, unsupervised, opportunity for recognition.

Impairment Limitations

				hands impaired:	*1*	*2*
blind	M1	balance	+	reaching	+	M2
low vision	M1	seizures	+	handling	M2	0
hearing	+	*aphasia:*		fingering	M2	0
speech	+	receptive	+	feeling	0	0
retardation	+	expressive	+	no hands	0	
memory	+	mixed	+			

impaired:

stooping	+	wheel chair	+	bed patient	+
kneeling	+	semi-ambulant	+	respiratory	+
crouching	+	Class III heart	+	*Energy Expenditure in*	
crawling	+	Class IV heart	+	*METS:* 1.2-2.0	

M1 may need assistance of a sighted person
M2 may need jig or fixture to hold materials

562 *Clothes and Dress Making* DD: 646.3-.4 LC: TT 500-560, HD 9942

Once home sewing was associated primarily with pinching pennies. While the economic advantages remain, greater sophistication in fabrics and design has raised the status of home sewing to a new level. Innovations and improvements by pattern companies have resulted in a greater range of available patterns from the very basic ("how-to-sew" patterns, simple enough for the most inexperienced novice) to very complex ("designer" patterns for the more practiced). Fabric prices vary similarily: the cost of attractive goods ranges from nominal to extravagant. These developments allow the seamstress to be both creative and practical. She can select design and fabric to fit her own needs and tastes in clothing. She can alter, modify, and design at will while improving her skill at the art. Lessons are given for a moderate fee, but many pick up the knack on their own, possibly with advice and assistance from the more experienced. This gives the individual a chance to produce on her own, but also makes possible sharing and interchange with others. Materials needed are more extensive, but at a price range flexible enough to fit most budgets.

570 *Wood and Metal Working Activities*

ENVIRONMENTAL FACTORS: indoor, no specific environment, modicum of space, equipment a major factor, equipment not necessarily at hand.

SOCIAL-PSYCHOLOGICAL FACTORS: aesthetic, utilitarian, creative, pre-patterned, concrete, individual effort, unstructured, supervised, unsupervised, opportunity for recognition.

Impairment Limitations

blind	M1	balance	M1	*hands impaired:*	1	2
low vision	M1	seizures	M1	reaching	M2	M2
hearing	+	*aphasia:*		handling	M2	M2
speech	+	receptive	+	fingering	M2	M2
retardation	+	expressive	+	feeling	M3	M3
memory	+	mixed	+	no hands	0	

impaired:						
stooping	+	wheel chair	M4	bed patient	M4	
kneeling	+	semi-ambulant	M4	respiratory	M5,	M6
crouching	+	Class III heart	M5	*Energy Expenditure in*		
crawling	+	Class IV heart	0	*METS:* 1.2-6.8		

M1 use hand tools rather than power tools
M2 hold objects in vise; use reaches, etc., if necessary
M3 watch out for hot objects, friction will heat up metal being cut or drilled
M4 may do bench activities
M5 use power tools instead of hand tools when possible
M6 install sawdust collector

573 Hand Tool Projects on Wood

Hand tool projects on wood: e.g., birdhouses, bookends, etc. DD: 648.082. LC: NK 9700-9799.

Although most woodworking projects can be done faster and often more accurately with power tools, small projects can be done with facility with hand tools. The skilled craftsman may achieve greater precision with chiseling and hand sanding than with machine routing and machine sanding.

There are innumerable sets of plans available for a great variety of small woodwork objects. In addition, many small objects can be custom designed for the artistic fulfillment of a particular house, or as a functional addition to a workshop or garage. Too many start woodworking as a hobby, make more birdhouses than can be given away to friends and relatives and, unable to think of anything else to make, drag themselves defeated back to watching TV. At the same time innumerable housewives yearn for an extra shelf in the kitchen.

Hand tools have greater portability and are indispensable where electric power is lacking as in camping, on boats, etc. Material costs may vary substantially. For an economy budget, wood scraps may be obtained from most lumber mills for nothing. Money invested in rare and expensive woods may yield finished products with exquisite grains and colors.

Uncontrolled epileptics and other accident-prone people may be well advised to choose hand tools over power tools.

574 Carpentry with Power Tools

Carpentry with power tools: e.g., lathe, circular saw, jig saw DD: 684.083. LC: TH 5601-5691.

Carpentry with power tools is a real joy, particularly to craftsmen previously limited to hand tools. So much can be accomplished so fast. An extremely wide range of tools and tool attachments are now available at moderate prices which permit most jobs to be done by power machinery. More time is now spent in setting up the machinery and attachments for the job at hand and storing attachments and materials for quick retrieval than in doing the actual job itself. Multiple purpose power tools, although representing less expensive initial investment, greatly increase the time required to change attachments and adjustments. This makes it more efficient to do several of the same kinds of jobs at once which leads to having several jobs going at once which requires more storage space, etc.

Machine tools require considerably more space than hand tools. Usually, the largest single unit of space is that required to cut a 4' × 8' piece of plywood on a circular saw.

For the hobbyist who does considerable work in his shop or a wide variety of work, the storage of wood supplies becomes a real problem. Having a sizeable stock of different kinds and sizes of wood greatly increases efficiency and lowers costs.

Large amounts of sawdust are produced by wood power tools and for individuals allergic to sawdust this is an unsuitable hobby unless they are willing to wear a dust protector or install dust collecting equipment.

577 Soldering and Welding DD: 682, 683 LC: TT 211, TS 225, TT 267

There seems to be no overt reason why some people prefer

working with wood and some with metal. These metalworking skills all involve using heat and burns are an ever present danger.

Close timing is an additional characteristic as the process involved must be performed at an exact point when the metal being worked on and/or the metal filler are exactly the right heat. This is difficult to describe in words or show in pictures. The experienced craftsman can help the apprentice with verbal corrections; the rest must be learned through experience.

Soldering is the simplest of the techniques and is useful for filling and decorating but has no load bearing capacity. Soldering joints on copper pipes is the most common household application.

Welding encompasses a wide range of skills and techniques, from simple cutting and brazing with a gas welder to welding aluminum with heliarc. Gas (oxy-acetylene) welding equipment is relatively inexpensive and extremely versatile. Gas welding is the easiest process to learn although a great deal of care is needed in handling the compressed gas. Arc welding is more difficult but is very useful when welding heavy plate.

Artistic welding has developed into a separate art form with almost unlimited potential for new designs in fountains, lawn decorations, mail box posts, etc. Junk metals may be used for some work which keeps the material costs within reasonable limits.

580 Handy Man Activities DD: 680 LC: TT 151

ENVIRONMENTAL FACTORS: indoor, outdoor, no specific environment, modicum of space, equipment a major factor, equipment not necessarily at hand.

SOCIAL-PSYCHOLOGICAL FACTORS: utilitarian, pre-patterned, concrete, individual effort, structured, unsupervised, opportunity for recognition.

Impairment Limitations

					hands impaired:	*1*	*2*
blind	S1	balance	M2		reaching	S4	S4
low vision	S2	seizures	M2		handling	M3	M4
hearing	+	*aphasia:*			fingering	M3	M4
speech	+	receptive	S3		feeling	M5	M5
retardation	S3	expressive	+		no hands	M4	
memory	M1	mixed	S3				

impaired:

stooping	S4	wheel chair	S4	bed patient	0
kneeling	S4	semi-ambulant	S4	respiratory	M6
crouching	S4	Class III heart	M6	*Energy Expenditure in*	
crawling	S4	Class IV heart	0	*METS:* 2-8	

M1 read instructions frequently and make notes of what has been done
M2 avoid climbing and work with power tools
M3 hold objects in vises, jigs and fixtures
M4 operate some small tools and brushes by holding in mouth or attached
    to head
M5 avoid hot objects
M6 light work at slow pace
S1 can do finishing and refinishing
S2 can work on large objects
S3 work on less technically complicated jobs
S4 can do bench work

Few activities have as many satisfying payoffs as handy man activities. They may add substantially to the net family income by reducing expenditures. They provide an outlet for the satisfactions of craftsmanship. Many of them satisfy aesthetic and creative needs. They contribute to a sense of camaraderie among fellow handy men, no matter how different their life styles in other respects.

There are innumerable books, magazines and pamphlets on practically all handy man activities. Before starting an activity, read about it in several sources. Frequently, a how-to-do-it process which cannot be clearly understood from reading one source is understandable after two or more explanations are read or diagrams inspected. The descriptions of materials given in some mail order catalogs may be very helpful.

Building and/or repairing the physical objects connected with his home helps the individual to recapture a feeling of understanding and controlling his physical environment. On the negative side, many handy activities are also a source of family friction. Wives may resent money spent on tools and materials from which no immediate return is visible. Repairs promised but delayed and jobs started and left incomplete, may violate some wives' concepts of a smooth running household. Storage room for tools and supplies becomes a problem. The smaller the residence, the greater the friction.

581 Simple Installation Activities

Simple installation activities: such as light bulbs, windows, screens, etc. DD: 681.83. LC: TK 9901.

These are necessary, usually regular, and sometimes seasonal activities with little psychic gain. They are chores which have to be done with negative implications if they are not done rather than positive implications if they are done. They do contribute to a sense of being a master of the environment in which we live, which for some is preferable to being subject to the whims of the janitor or maintenance man in those apartment houses where these services are provided.

582 Complex Installation Activities

Complex installation activities: such as tiles, carpets, paneling, plastering, drywall. DD: 698, 698.9. LC: TP 837-9.

Since the results of these installations are highly visible, there is substantial satisfaction from having a workmanship-like job to show friends and brag about discreetly. In some cases, choosing the colors, type of materials and texture of the finish is an aesthetically pleasing experience.

A fair degree of craftsmanship is required for these activities because little correction is possible once the materials have been cut. This requires precise measurements and, for beginners, a great deal of checking and rechecking. Better start in a closet where mistakes can become skeletons and kept out of sight!

583 Interior and Exterior House Painting DD: 698.1 LC: TT 300-380

Few things produce as much aesthetic satisfaction and sense of accomplishment with as little skill. It also makes the largest contribution to the net family income because the proportion of labor costs savings in relation to material costs are so high. Outside painting, if it includes thorough caulking as a prerequisite, is a major money saver over the long run by reducing house deterioration.

The choice of colors and combination of colors offer a chance for highly visible artistic expression. This is one activity in which individuals with only one functionally useable arm remaining have relatively little handicap.

584 *Repairing, Varnishing, Staining, etc., of Furniture, Woodwork, etc.* DD: 684.1-.2 LC: TT 300-380

The time consuming nature of these activities makes the cost of purchasing this work commercially almost prohibitive, so that substantial savings for the family net income are realized through this hobby. It is particularly suitable for individuals who enjoy producing an aesthetically enjoyable finished product. Refinishing is also highly suited to those with the use of only one arm remaining.

590 *Miscellaneous Craft Activities* DD: 745 LC: TT, NK

ENVIRONMENTAL FACTORS: indoor, outdoor, no specific environment, modicum of space, unlimited space, equipment a major factor, equipment not necessarily at hand.

SOCIAL-PSYCHOLOGICAL FACTORS: aesthetic, creative, concrete, individual effort, unstructured, unsupervised, opportunity for recognition.

Impairment Limitations

blind	0	balance	S1	*hands impaired:*	*1*	*2*
low vision	S1	seizures	M1	reaching	+	S1
hearing	+	*aphasia:*		handling	+	S1
speech	+	receptive	+	fingering	+	S1
retardation	+	expressive	+	feeling	M1	M1
memory	+	mixed	+	no hands	0	
impaired:						
stooping	+	wheel chair	S1	bed patient	S1	
kneeling	+	semi-ambulant	S1	respiratory	+	
crouching	+	Class III heart	S1	*Energy Expenditure in*		
crawling	+	Class IV heart	M2	*METS:* 1.2-6.8		

S1   everything except kite flying
M1   protect against hot wax in candlemaking
M2   limited to lightest materials

There seems to be a rebirth of interest in craft activities as recreational pursuits. With good reason, it might be said that the Counter-Industrial Revolution has begun, for much of the craft activity is in reply to the abundance of the ready-made. Sociological implications aside, this development is very useful for purposes of directed avocational activities. Books on how-to-do-it, materials to do it with, even where-to-get-it catalogs are in abundance. Most craftsmen would vouch that the internal satisfaction is reward enough for the external product, but many crafts have the additional advantage of being easily marketable, beginner's work no exception. Results are immediate enough to provide further incentive. These crafts, as a medium of personal expression, might help someone say more than he can in words. Most craft activities are flexible enough to adapt to a variety of mental and physical abilities.

591 Collage and Decoupage DD: 746 LC: NK 9315

A collage expresses an idea by means of a combination of smaller ideas. That is, in making a collage, one pastes together all manner of cuttings from paper and each cutting contributes to the theme of the whole. These are very imaginative and very subjective creations and may be done using a variety of materials, most of which are very common, even relatively insignificant except when used in this context. They then take on important connotations, may be interpreted at many different levels of meaning, and add to the subtle complexity of the theme.

A collage is an exercise in imaginative use of simple materials. Often the most fun is in looking for the appropriate materials, e.g., rummaging through magazines in search of pictures which will lend themselves to the desired creation. In making a collage, one visualizes the desired result, then judges the effectiveness of the means of expression. There is a certain talent required in judging spatial relations, color and form, evaluation of the composition as a whole. However, these considerations should not be allowed to interfere with the relative freedom enjoyed in making collages. Too often artistic expression is hampered in the timid or hesitant for fear of not meeting up with arbitrary standards. Collages may be an excellent form of encouraging self-expression.

593 *Mosaics* DD: 748.5 LC: NK 5430, NK 8500

Working with mosaic is a test of patience and creative design. This is close, slow, and painstaking work. While it may be an excellent device for those with an abundance of leisure time, progress on the work may be slower than some would wish. It would be better reserved for those who care for intricately worked designs. Materials may be glass, marble or even paper. Designs may be imitative or original. One outgrowth might be an interest in art history, possibly a specialized interest in Roman or Byzantine mosaic work.

594 *Fountain Construction* DD: 714 LC: NA 9400-9425

Fountains may be constructed of concrete, copper, steel, aluminum, brick, or stone and an almost infinite number of designs are possible. Small relatively inexpensive submersible pumps may be used. The least complex outdoor fountains can be made of poured concrete and junk materials, such as an old auto fender turned upside down, may be used to form pools. The pipes and other metal parts are fabricated by soldering, brazing, or welding. Small indoor fountains can be made of light copper tubing which can be bent by hand and soldered. Fountains may be lighted at night with revolving and/or changing colored lights. Because of the contrast, fountains are particularly satisfying in hot, dry climates.

610 *Photography* DD: 770 LC: TR

ENVIRONMENTAL FACTORS: indoor, outdoor, specialized environment and/or climate, modicum of space, equipment a major factor, equipment not necessarily at hand.

SOCIAL-PSYCHOLOGICAL FACTORS: aesthetic, creative, abstract, concrete, group effort, individual effort, unstructured, unsupervised, opportunity for recognition.

Impairment Limitations

blind	S1	balance	M2	*hands impaired:*	*1*	*2*
low vision	S1	seizures	+	reaching	M2	M2
hearing	+	*aphasia:*		handling	M2	0
speech	+	receptive	+	fingering	M2	0
retardation	+	expressive	+	feeling	+	+
memory	M1	mixed	+	no hands	0	

impaired:

stooping	+	wheel chair	+	bed patient	S2
kneeling	+	semi-ambulant	M2	respiratory	M3
crouching	+	Class III heart	+	*Energy Expenditure in*	
crawling	+	Class IV heart	S2	*METS:* 1.3-4.4	

M1 makes notes of where/when pictures taken, lens speed, aperture reading, etc.

M2 use tripod or limit to table top photography

M3 avoid if irritated by acetic acid (vinegar)

S1 darkroom only

S2 with these limitations, individuals can still take pictures of indoor objects around them, outside shots through windows, posed pictures of friends and still life which is arranged for them

The challenge of photography lies in the mastery of equipment to produce an image which is artistically pleasing and creatively expressive. Making a picture is as valid a means of expressing oneself as is painting or writing. Whether you take pictures with a Kodak instamatic or a Nikon, the concept of re-creating a moment captured with the mechanical extension of the human eye remains the same.

An artistic sense of balanced composition, a good eye for images, and a fairly steady hand are definite assets for making satisfactory pictures. With guidance almost anyone can come up with a decent photograph.

Photography can be undertaken on different scales. The degree of personal satisfaction one derives from photography depends directly on how much effort he puts into it. The beginner can learn without too much difficulty how to operate an automatic camera. As one gains more confidence in himself and his eye, he might want to have more control over his settings.

While the physical and creative process of making a picture is a solitary task, the interaction in photography comes when photographers share their knowledge and their work. Clubs can be organized around this interest thereby enabling photographers to share costs, equipment and encouragement.

The chemical processing of negatives and prints can be divided into separate tasks, the mechanics of which require varying degrees of manual dexterity, a precise sense of timing, sound judgment and, for printing especially, a sharp eye.

Development of negatives is a process carried on almost totally in the dark. Success depends mainly on the ability to handle film by feel rather than by sight, careful attention to proper method, and accurate timing for each procedure.

After the negatives have been developed and dried, the printing of a picture is executed in semi-darkness and involves the use of an enlarging machine. Competence in this area can be acquired through general instruction, but is achieved most through constant practice. After a picture has gone through all the chemicals, it must be thrown into a washing bin and then placed in a dryer. Both steps are largely uncomplicated and with minimal training, anyone can become proficient at either task.

Film processing is expensive no matter how primitive the photo-lab. Another drawback to film processing is that, separated from the creative elements of camera work, it tends to become tedious and mechanical. While there is some personal gratification attached to competent technical skill, it is not a rewarding activity for someone who requires recognition as a motivating force. It is generally an anonymous job, with praise for the finished print going to the one who snapped the shutter. On the other hand, work in the photo-lab would encourage cooperation among aspiring technicians and would also inspire self-confidence through development of accurate judgment.

620 *Drawing and Printing Activities* DD: 740, 769 LC: NC-Z 116-265

ENVIRONMENTAL FACTORS: indoor, outdoor, no specific environment, modicum of space, equipment a major factor, equipment not necessarily at hand.

SOCIAL-PSYCHOLOGICAL FACTORS: aesthetic, utilitarian, creative, pre-patterned, concrete, individual effort, structured, unstructured, unsupervised, opportunity for recognition.

Impairment Limitations

blind	0	balance	+	*hands impaired:*	1	2
low vision	M1	seizures	+	reaching	+	+
hearing	+	*aphasia:*		handling	M2	M3
speech	+	receptive	+	fingering	M2	M3
retardation	S1	expressive	+	feeling	+	+
memory	+	mixed	+	no hands	M3	

impaired:

stooping	+	wheel chair	+	bed patient	+
kneeling	+	semi-ambulant	+	respiratory	+
crouching	+	Class III heart	+	*Energy Expenditure in*	
crawling	+	Class IV heart	+	*METS:* 1.4-3.2	

M1 no fine detail
M2 hold work in jig or thumb tack down
M3 may draw holding pencil, pen or brush in mouth or attached to head
S1 can do etching and stenciling

These activities are specialized groups within the general categories of graphic arts and visual arts. The graphic arts are considered to be representational art forms, i.e., they are concerned more with accurate reproduction of forms than with the creation of those forms. This would suggest that, in working with these media, one need not be original to the extent that other art forms may require. And yet originality and creativity may be expressed—one's own attitude or mood or conceptions may be conveyed in the designs or styles used. In this respect, graphic arts may be every bit as demanding as other visual arts, which are more generally considered to be expressive of personal creativity. Nonetheless, if we hold to the definition of graphic arts as skillful reproduction of what has already been created, by contrast we might define visual arts as the skillful use of individual perceptions to add new dimensions to what has already been created. Thus, what distinguishes Cezanne's still life from Picasso's still life has to do with the personal expressions of the artist.

Although these activities are classified according to what seems to be a natural separation, this division is not to be considered absolute. All of the activities require in greater or lesser degrees a sense of the aesthetic, of artistic principles—sense of balance, proportion and color, of perspective and form in space. On the whole, successful results in these activities are not without much slow-going tedious work. Patience and the will to persevere are just as important as artistic talent.

625 *Cartoon and Caricature* DD: 741.5 LC: NC 1300-1763

Cartoons and caricatures are visual editorials on characters and characteristics of a society. As comments on the times, they may be bitterly satirical, derisive and mocking, mildly amusing, or poignantly sorrowful. Whatever the tone, the cartoon or caricature is successful through the simplicity and directness of its expression. A sharp, inventive mind with an incisive grasp of political or social conditions and/or individuals who represent those conditions fulfills half the requirements of a good cartoonist or caricaturist. Ability to translate thought into simple yet effective visual expression supplies the other half. This ability includes understanding of technical principles of form, line, color and composition.

Cartoons and caricatures enjoy extensive popularity, although they are appreciated less by the victim of the attack. Political and social minorities execute some of the more bitter pieces. There is no guarantee that visual expression sweetens bitter sentiments. It may be argued that this is not the most socially constructive of activities. It certainly is a very powerful and influential one.

Cartooning on a more popular scale takes the form of the comic strip. Generally these are milder, more humorous interpretations of the culture. Because they normally engage in less direct and biting attacks, there is less risk of offense and greater chance of social approbation.

626 *Clothes Design* DD: 687.1 LC: TT 500-560

Clothing design as an avocational activity will probably enjoy its greatest appeal among those who already are devoted home sewers. Once the principles of sewing techniques—pattern design, construction, fabric and color coordination—are adequately understood, the experienced seamstress can muster her understanding into working designs of her own creation. The crucial factor in success—whether the seamstress is formally instructed or self-taught—is actual practice. Only working through different stages and types of patterns will provide the necessary background to individual creative endeavors. One of the advantages of this activity is the chance it gives for personal expression in a creative and concrete way. The results are tangible; mistakes aren't irreparable. Benefits are the praise, admiration, even envy of others. Since the seamstress often shares the role of housewife, which too often is a role of unrelieved drudgery, this activity can prove invaluable in restoring her sense of creativity.

630 *Painting Activities* DD: 750-751 LC: ND

ENVIRONMENTAL FACTORS: indoor, outdoor, no specific environment, modicum of space, requires little or no equipment, equipment not necessarily at hand.

SOCIAL-PSYCHOLOGICAL FACTORS: aesthetic, creative, abstract, individual effort, unstructured, unsupervised, opportunity for recognition.

Impairment Limitations

						hands impaired:	*1*	*2*
blind	0		balance	+		reaching	+	M2
low vision	M1		seizures	+		handling	+	M2
hearing	+		*aphasia:*			fingering	+	M2
speech	+		receptive	+		feeling	+	+
retardation	+		expressive	+		no hands	M2	
memory	+		mixed	+				

impaired:								
stooping	+		wheel chair	+		bed patient	+	
kneeling	+		semi-ambulant	+		respiratory	+	
crouching	+		Class III heart	+		*Energy Expenditure in*		
crawling	+		Class IV heart	+		*METS:* 1.4-3.2		

M1 no fine detail
M2 may hold brush in mouth or attached to head; may paint with feet
There is an Association of Handicapped Artists Inc., in Buffalo, N.Y.

Painting activities are creative visual expressions. That they are an outlet for expression of ideas ties them to other arts—music and literature. That their appeal is expressly to the visual is what distinguishes them. The "message" of the painting is conveyed by the particular choice and combination of form, color and subject. The artist is aware of the symbolic message of these choices. The skilled artist working within a tradition is aware of and works with the wide ranges of connotation for the symbols. This genius, combined with highly skilled craftsmanship is what makes a great artist.

Quite naturally, not all those who attempt to paint are going to reach this level of art. Quite possibly, many of those who try are going to glean at least some measure of artistic sensitivity or an appreciation that painting may involve much more than attempts at reduplication of a subject. Many of the aesthetic questions involved may be of no concern to the amateur. For him, the question of importance will be the pleasure he derives from the created object and the sense of his participation in its creation.

Painting appeals to the individual. All the steps in its conception and execution—choice of method, subject, theme, color, form—are his own. The responsibility for its success or failure to be all it was intended are also his own. Depending upon how intensely the artist himself is involved with his creation, painting may become more than just a spare time hobby, in which case difficulties, shortcomings in the execution of the work, may produce, instead of alleviate, difficulties.

640 Sculpture and Carving Activities DD: 736 LC: NB

ENVIRONMENTAL FACTORS: indoor, outdoor, no specific environment, specialized environment and/or climate, modicum of space, requires little or no equipment, equipment a major factor, equipment not necessarily at hand.

SOCIAL-PSYCHOLOGICAL FACTORS: aesthetic, creative, concrete, individual effort, unstructured, unsupervised, opportunity for recognition.

Impairment Limitations

blind	+	balance	+	*hands impaired:*	*1*	*2*
low vision	+	seizures	+	reaching	+	0
hearing	+	*aphasia:*		handling	S1	0
speech	+	receptive	+	fingering	S1	0
retardation	+	expressive	+	feeling	+	M1
memory	+	mixed	+	no hands	0	

impaired:					
stooping	+	wheel chair	+	bed patient	S1
kneeling	+	semi-ambulant	+	respiratory	M2
crouching	+	Class III heart	+	*Energy Expenditure in*	
crawling	+	Class IV heart	S1	*METS:* 1.4-5	

M1 protect against cuts and bruises
M2 install dust removal equipment if working with stone
S1   can carve soft objects: clay, putty, soap, wax

Sculpture is a visual expression in three-dimensional form. As fine art, it is the physical representation of an idea. As commercial art, sculpture may suffer in its translation to lowest common denominator tastes. Like most other artistic forms, sculpture calls for both a creative mind and a skilled hand. One works at once in both the abstract and the concrete. In the abstract, one is concerned with balance, proportion, shape, form, mass and volume and their relation to space, and light patterns. The overall concern is how to work all these elements into a composition. In the concrete, one needs an understanding of the materials—their properties and textures, what they are and are not suited for. Other considerations are some techniques proper to sculpture—armatures, carving, casting, glazing.

Most often formal instruction is suggested for beginners. Art courses are also recommended. Neither is essential, especially for forms of sculpture like wax and soap carving or clay and putty modeling. One should note, too, that sculpture can be very physically demanding. Many of the types of sculpture listed here might be pursued at a less formal level of technical skill and artistic intent and at the same time be quite valuable in illustrating the relation between the two.

Perhaps the most important aspect is the possible opportunity to work out one's imaginings and concepts and visions into a tangible reality. The medium chosen may be expressive of the person's temperament. The person without the patience to persevere through a whole wood carving can use wire instead. Working with different forms may give the person a better sense of materials—why one can do this with wire, but not with wood. Having developed this sense, the next step might be the choice of the best medium to convey the preconceived form.

650 Drama Activities

ENVIRONMENTAL FACTORS: indoor, no specific environment, modicum of space, requires little or no equipment, equipment normally at hand, equipment not necessarily at hand.

SOCIAL-PSYCHOLOGICAL FACTORS: aesthetic, creative, pre-patterned, abstract, group effort, individual effort, structured, unstructured, supervised, unsupervised, opportunity for recognition.

Impairment Limitations

blind	S1	balance	+	*hands impaired:*	*1*	*2*
low vision	S1	seizures	+	reaching	S3	S3
hearing	S2	*aphasia:*		handling	S3	S3
speech	S2	receptive	0	fingering	S3	S3
retardation	+	expressive	S2	feeling	+	+
memory	0	mixed	0	no hands	S3	

impaired:

stooping	+	wheel chair	+	bed patient	S4
kneeling	+	semi-ambulant	+	respiratory	+
crouching	+	Class III heart	M1	*Energy Expenditure in*	
crawling	+	Class IV heart	S4,M1	*METS:* 1.4-3.0	

M1 if the situation does not precipitate excessive psychological stress in the
   individual
S1 limited to oral expression
S2 everything but oral expression
S3 everything but operating complex puppets, marionettes and stage
   equipment
S4 jokes, storytelling, etc.

655 *Psychodramas, Sociodramas, Role Playing* DD: 792.2 LC: RC 489

Different definitions of these activities are offered by different authors and there is considerable overlap in the meanings of
each. Consequently, the descriptions given below are rough guidelines rather than conceptually clear statements.

Role playing is acting according to a role other than the role
one normally assumes. This can lead to dynamic insights into the
problems faced by others and why they believe and behave the
way they do. It may be a useful conflict resolution device and has
been used in this manner in family therapy. If used as a parlor
game, roles should be chosen which are not too threatening to
the participants and no one should be urged to participate if he
feels uncomfortable in doing so.

Psychodrama is used as a therapeutic instrument under the
supervision of a psychotherapist to help patients gain more insight into their own behavior and to help the therapist better
understand how the patient reacts in social situations. Carefully
selected and trained volunteers may help as props by enacting

such roles as the patient's father, mother, spouse, boss, etc. Psychodramas should *not* be used as a parlor game, since it can be traumatic to emotionally unstable people.

Sociodrama, in contrast to psychodrama, is less concerned with the problems of an individual actor and more concerned with the attitudes and behavior of a group of people in a prescribed structured situation. This has been used in research on attitudes and prejudices to collect information not easily obtained by direct questioning. As a parlor game, it may help the participants gain new insights into attitudes and beliefs of others.

657 Play Direction and Production DD: 792.023 LC: PN 1660-1691

For the talented individual who has had some experience with drama, play direction and production can provide excellent creative outlets.

The director of a dramatic production is charged with the responsibility of coordinating the efforts of the individual performers. His is the task of synthesizing the diverse talents of the actors and actresses and molding their performances into a unified whole. The director need not have outstanding dramatic talent, but he must have an understanding of the dramatic processes, and he must, more importantly, have a real knack for handling people. The director has to convince the performers that they should do what he wants them to do, at the same time making them believe that in so doing they are only doing what they really wanted to do all along, and are only responding to their own creative impulses. The director must also be able to help the performers get along with each other, since a smooth production isn't possible without smooth interaction among the performers.

The producer's job is to oversee the whole show—not only the dramatic efforts of the performers and director, but such details as scenery, ticket sales, lighting, choreography, publicity, and financing. The final responsibility for having the show go on is usually the producer's. He needs to have all the understanding that the director has of what is actually going on, plus organizational talent and an inexhaustible supply of patience and tact. It is even more important that the producer be talented at dealing with people than that the director have this ability, for the producer has not only to coordinate the efforts of the actors and actresses and director, but he must also be able to handle playwrights, flat painters, and purchasing agents.

660 Dance Activities

ENVIRONMENTAL FACTORS: indoor, outdoor, no specific environment, modicum of space, unlimited space, requires little or no equipment, equipment normally at hand.

SOCIAL-PSYCHOLOGICAL FACTORS: aesthetic, creative, pre-patterned, concrete, group effort, individual effort, structured, unstructured, supervised, unsupervised, opportunity for recognition.

Impairment Limitations

blind	M1	balance	0	*hands impaired:*	*1*	*2*
low vision	+	seizures	+	reaching	S1	S1
hearing	+	*aphasia:*		handling	+	+
speech	+	receptive	+	fingering	+	+
retardation	+	expressive	+	feeling	+	+
memory	M1	mixed	+	no hands	S1	

impaired:

stooping	+	wheel chair	0	bed patient	0
kneeling	+	semi-ambulant	0	respiratory	M2
crouching	+	Class III heart	M2	*Energy Expenditure in*	
crawling	+	Class IV heart	0	*METS:* 5.5-10	

M1 dependent on partner for guidance
M2 limited to slow pace for short periods
S1 limited in dances involving holding partner

662 Popular Dancing DD: 793.3 LC: GV 1783

Popular dancing is essentially a social activity. Currently, dancing done among young people to popular music is highly unstructured. The primary requirements for success are a sense of rhythm and a lack of inhibitions, although an understanding and friendly partner can also be helpful.

The primary benefits of this activity are the social contacts it brings about and the increased self-confidence of the dancer who learns that he can express himself through dancing. Initial self-consciousness is unavoidable, but if the individual is unduly apprehensive about the picture he is going to present on the dance floor, a few informal lessons in a private setting might be helpful.

663 *Ballroom Dancing* DD: 793.33 LC: GV 1751

Ballroom dancing (the waltz, fox trot, etc.) is generally a bit more structured than popular dancing. Although the accomplished dancer may sometimes add his own flourishes, there are basic steps to be followed in most of these dances.

The basic steps of most ballroom dancing are fairly simple and easy to master. One can become a fairly good dancer with relatively little practice. The subtleties of the art, however, increase with practice; many years can be spent improving technique.

As in many dance activities, the chief benefit of ballroom dancing lies in its social aspect. It is impossible to waltz without a partner; cooperation between partners is essential to success. Dancing of this kind has an aura of elegance about it which is not present in other types of dancing; although the relative formality of the situation may cause some people to freeze, it is more likely to bring out hidden gallantries. Middle-aged and older people who take up this activity are apt to be more comfortable with it than they would be with many other types of dancing; people in these age groups tend to worry about losing their dignity in public, and ballroom dancing is usually acceptable to them.

Physically, ballroom dancing is an excellent rhythmic activity, including many levels of exertion and skill. Most ballroom dancing is done to music which has strong points of rhythmic emphasis, which is helpful to those who do not have an extremely well-developed sense of rhythm.

664 *Square Dancing* DD: 793.34 LC: GV 1763

Square dancing, involving eight people (four couples) in simple to intricate patterns of dance movements, is a distinctly social affair. In western type square dancing, more people and couples tend to be in motion at the same time, greatly increasing the complexity of the movements and making greater demands on the dancers. There is a considerable range of role performance possible. Beginners are pushed, pulled, coaxed through the movements; old timers add individual embellishments. Role performance varies with age; the young may perform the dance with incredible vigor; the old may shuffle through it. Square dancing may also be considered a forerunner of sensitivity training. Each dancer is systematically brought into physical contact with the other seven dancers in the square. Memory, spatial relations, and a sense of community with other people are required. Although square dance records with calls are available, the services of a professional or amateur caller are highly desirable, since a live caller can pace the activity to the level of the dancers.

670 Music Activities

ENVIRONMENTAL FACTORS: indoor, outdoor, no specific environment, modicum of space, equipment a major factor, equipment not necessarily at hand.

SOCIAL-PSYCHOLOGICAL FACTORS: aesthetic, creative, pre-patterned, abstract, concrete, group effort, individual effort, structured, unstructured, supervised, unsupervised, opportunity for recognition, little opportunity for recognition.

Impairment Limitations

						hands impaired:	*1*	*2*
blind	+		balance	+		reaching	S1	S2
low vision	+		seizures	+		handling	S1	S2
hearing	0		*aphasia:*			fingering	S1	S2
speech	+		receptive	M1		feeling	S1	S2
retardation	+		expressive	+		no hands	S2	
memory	M1		mixed	+				

impaired:

stooping	+	wheel chair	+	bed patient	S4
kneeling	+	semi-ambulant	+	respiratory	S5
crouching	+	Class III heart	+	*Energy Expenditure in*	
crawling	+	Class IV heart	S3	*METS:* 2.0-2.5	

M1 cannot memorize scores
S1 limited to singing, conducting, writing and instruments which can be played with one hand
S2 limited to singing, writing and foot-operated drum
S3 limited to writing
S4 limited to writing and small instruments: mouth organ, jewsharp, recorder
S5 may be restricted in playing wind instruments

672 Solo Singing and/or Instrument Playing DD: 781.3061 LC: MT 870, MT 885, ML 462

The delight in physical response to music comes to play as a motivational factor in the desire to master more specialized and complex forms of music. The basic sense of what makes music is intensified by the understanding of how the instrument—vocal, stringed, wind, or percussion—makes music. Except for the rare musical prodigy, a structured, supervised setting is needed. The social nature of the setting shifts to the individual, just as the discipline and motivation needed to persist must be his. If he perseveres through the often tedious, seemingly fruitless periods of practice, the rewards, too, the personal satisfaction and delight at being able in some way to create music, are his.

675 Playing in Musical Groups

Playing in musical groups: e.g. bands, orchestras, etc. DD: 785.7, 784.1-.3, 785.4. LC: MT 893, MT 88, MT 733, ML 1300-1354, ML 1200-1251, M900-949.

The combining of one's musical skills with those of others brings the "group" element back into play. One plays one's own part, but coordinates, blends, contrasts it with the parts of others. The whole of the music equals the sum of its many parts and is as good or bad as the many. Yours is not the complete music, nor without yours is the music complete. For those not equal to the challenge of solo performances, whether musically or psychologically, group playing arranges a more comfortable display of talents. In the same vein, informal, as opposed to formal, performances comfortably allow for less than perfect mastery.

680 Writing Activities 808.001-.709 LC: Z 40-115

ENVIRONMENTAL FACTORS: indoor, outdoor, no specific environment, modicum of space, requires little or no equipment, equipment normally at hand.

SOCIAL-PSYCHOLOGICAL FACTORS: aesthetic, creative, abstract, concrete, individual effort, structured, unstructured, unsupervised, opportunity for recognition.

Impairment Limitations

blind	M1	balance	+	*hands impaired:*	1	2
low vision	+	seizures	+	reaching	+	+
hearing	+	*aphasia:*		handling	+	M2
speech	+	receptive	0	fingering	+	M2
retardation	0	expressive	0	feeling	+	M2
memory	+	mixed	0	no hands	M2	

impaired:

stooping	+	wheel chair	+	bed patient	+
kneeling	+	semi-ambulant	+	respiratory	+
crouching	+	Class III heart	+	*Energy Expenditure in*	
crawling	+	Class IV heart	+	*METS:* 1.4	

M1 can dictate or type
M2 can dictate

Writing activities on almost every level—doggerel verse, friendly letter, or art—demand the writer to commit himself to the blank page in front of him and overcome it. The good writer wants to fill the page with the clearest, most perceptive thoughts he can produce, and for him the act of writing is a challenge of the highest order.

Whether the final product is one of wit and whimsy or of passionate earnestness, the act of writing summons within a person a strong feeling of commitment to his words and to those persons for whom he is writing. A writer in the act of writing works at his highest levels of intelligence and concentration; he brings together discipline and spontaneity, two seemingly opposed attributes without which good writing cannot come into existence.

The important fact is that this commitment, this intelligence, this discipline and spontaneity are present to some degree in every kind of writing. The thrill of harnessing a thought into words on paper is one which awaits anyone, of whatever abilities, who takes time to do it.

An aside: to write anything meaningful the writer must overcome within himself the basic human fear of self-recognition, the fear which leads us to compromise ourselves and repress those feelings which might, if given free rein, call for drastic changes in our ways of living and acting. A poet of the American Midwest said he only wanted to tell people things they already knew. Such honesty should stand as an ideal for any writing endeavor.

681 *Letter Writing* DD: 808.6 LC: PE 1479-1481, BJ 2100-2115

Letter writing is one of the most creative and fulfilling kinds of writing because it has the least restricting structure of all. A letter writer can call into play any element of communication, verbal and visual, without fear of violating form or literary protocol. Letter writing as a key vehicle of friendship should encourage the writer to express himself as freely as possible. People with a desperate need for companionship, including those with confining disabilities, might turn to letter writing (perhaps with pen pals in similar situations) as an important social outlet and morale booster.

688 *Poetry* DD: 808.1-.3 LC: PN 1040-1059, PN 1101, PN 1660-1707, PN 3355-3385

Short stories, novels, dramas and poetry allow the writer to venture as far as he can into his and others' emotions. As mentioned above, such serious writing presents a formidable challenge to the writer, but he can approach the truth of life itself if he's willing to exert the effort. Such creative writing, of course, can be undertaken as a pleasant diversion, too, in the form of light parody or melodrama. But all forms of creative writing require a degree of sensitivity to life. For those who have the sensitivity, originality, and skill to write creatively, leisure time can acquire a whole new meaning, from merely an interval between work periods to a continuing voyage of artistic exploration and discovery.

690 *Miscellaneous Art and Music Activities*

ENVIRONMENTAL FACTORS: indoor, outdoor, no specific environment, modicum of space, equipment a major factor, equipment not necessarily at hand.

SOCIAL-PSYCHOLOGICAL FACTORS: aesthetic, creative, abstract, group effort, individual effort, unstructured, opportunity for recognition, unsupervised.

110 *Avocational Activities*

Impairment Limitations

blind	0	balance	M2	*hands impaired:*	*1*	*2*
low vision	0	seizures	+	reaching	+	0
speech	+	*aphasia:*		handling	+	0
hearing	+	receptive	+	fingering	+	0
retardation	0	expressive	+	feeling	+	+
memory	M1	mixed	+	no hands	0	

impaired:

stooping	M3	wheel chair	+	bed patient	0
kneeling	M3	semi-ambulant	M2	respiratory	+
crouching	M3	Class III heart	+	*Energy Expenditure in*	
crawling	M3	Class IV heart	0	*METS:* 1.4-3	

M1 require extensive note taking to recall sequence of movie making
M2 use tripod for camera
M3 may require special camera adaptations for angle shots, etc.

691 Film Production DD: 778.5 LC: PN 1997.85, PN 1992-1999

The film is another form of visual art. Behind a film is the idea the "author" wishes to communicate. In this respect, film production is extremely subjective and allows for much creativity on the part of the film maker. However, the actual production of this visual design entails a rigorous series of steps whose execution demands manual and visual skills. In this respect, film production is logical and analytical and calls for much discipline on the part of the film maker.

The most basic requirement is familiarity with and ability in handling a camera and camera equipment. Beyond knowing enough to take a good picture, this means also knowing the how, when and why of film and film speeds, exposure, filters and lights. Taking it a step further, this may also entail printing and re-touching. This understanding of the technical aspects will come to play in straight filming, but it may also be of special use in filming to produce special effects.

Beyond the skill in the actual filming is the required skill in composition. The film producer must construct the logical sequence of the action, taking into account the timing and rhythm of movement in order to achieve continuity. He must have a sense of the desired whole and a sense of how the individual scenes are to fit into that whole. He has decided on a theme and his attitude towards that theme, and must employ techniques suited to both. This part of the filming focuses on his originality as well as his powers of judgment.

The film producer can play a very influential role. He may creatively express his emotions, attitudes or criticisms into an effective and compelling visual statement. Or he may pursue films purely for aesthetics, experimenting with various techniques to produce certain visual effects.

Although it may sound like quite a complicated project, film making is not beyond the powers of the ordinary. Film making has been taught to school children, who picked it up with very little trouble. Films need not be on the Cecil B. De Mille level of spectacular in order to be good films. Their relative youth as artistic form and their flexibility make them fertile ground for artistic endeavor.

710 Radio Listening

ENVIRONMENTAL FACTORS: indoor, no specific environment, modicum of space, equipment a major factor, equipment normally at hand.

SOCIAL-PSYCHOLOGICAL FACTORS: aesthetic, utilitarian, pre-patterned, abstract, concrete, individual effort, structured, supervised, little opportunity for recognition.

Impairment Limitations

blind	+	balance	+	*hands impaired:*	*1*	*2*
low vision	+	seizures	+	reaching	+	+
hearing	0	*aphasia:*		handling	+	M1
speech	+	receptive	+	fingering	+	M1
retardation	+	expressive	+	feeling	+	+
memory	+	mixed	+	no hands	M1	

impaired:

stooping	+	wheel chair	+	bed patient	+
kneeling	+	semi-ambulant	+	respiratory	+
crouching	+	Class III heart	+	*Energy Expenditure in*	
crawling	+	Class IV heart	+	*METS:* 1.2-1.4	

M1 need push button tuning and push button on-off switch

712 Interview and Talk Shows, Telephone Forums DD: 791.447
LC: TK 6570.A-Z

In this age of alienation in which the individual frequently
feels that he has little interaction with important events going on
and no control over important decisions made, these shows provide an important link whereby the listener has a chance to talk
back, to question the interpretations which have been given him
through the mass media, to argue, to disagree, to persuade and
symbolically at least, to control his social environment by expressing his opinion over a medium through which it will be
heard by a substantial number of people. This is one way of maintaining some dimension of participatory democracy in a mass
society and using technology to unite rather than fracture interaction in the society. Because the master of ceremonies or inter-
viewer can cross-examine speakers, the weaknesses and biases in
the speaker's presentation may be revealed. Telephone forums
offer an excellent opportunity for homebound individuals to participate in the larger social world.

713 News Commentaries DD: 791.447 LC: TK 6570.A-Z

These commentaries are useful in helping the listener to
understand the news better, providing the commentator actually
has more knowledge and information. Commentaries are more
helpful when two or more commentators discuss the same topic
so that the views of one may be evaluated against the views of
another. It also helps for the listener to have maps at hand if the
commentary involves geographical background as, for instance,
in evaluating military actions and strategies. Understanding commentaries on economic events may be aided by having at hand
graphs and charts of economic activities. If a listener listens to a
commentator regularly, the wise listener will list the commentator's prejudices and biases so that he can correct them.

720 Television Watching DD: 791.45 LC: TK 6630, HE 8690-
8699

ENVIRONMENTAL FACTORS: indoor, no specific environment,
modicum of space, equipment a major factor, equipment normally at hand.

SOCIAL-PSYCHOLOGICAL FACTORS: aesthetic, utilitarian, pre-patterned, concrete, individual effort, structured, supervised, little opportunity for recognition.

Impairment Limitations

blind	M1	balance	+	*hands impaired:*	*1*	*2*
low vision	+	seizures	+	reaching	+	+
hearing	M2	*aphasia:*		handling	+	M3
speech	+	receptive	+	fingering	+	M3
retardation	+	expressive	+	feeling	+	+
memory	+	mixed	+	no hands	M1	

impaired:					
stooping	+	wheel chair	+	bed patient	+
kneeling	+	semi-ambulant	+	respiratory	+
crouching	+	Class III heart	+	*Energy Expenditure in*	
crawling	+	Class IV heart	+	*METS:* 1.2-1.4	

M1 can listen
M2 can see but not hear
M3 need push button tuning and push button on-off switch

TV watching is so commonplace that the many nuances of intelligent and purposeful versus aimless watching are overlooked. How and what the consumer watches may determine whether he uses the TV as an instrument of personal development or succumbs to it as an audio-visual drug.

All programs can be usefully subjected to a variety of analyses. Here are some of the things to look for:

1. What major values in American society is the program reflecting?
2. In programs reflecting values of society, are the actors, speakers, or other participants involved projecting reasoned and intelligent views or reinforcing unthinking or deeply rooted biases?
3. What models or symbols are presented? Are these presented as desirable or undesirable?
4. How technically adequate are the presentations in the following dimensions: analysis of social events; psychological characterizations; acting; neutrality of the host on talk shows and panel discussions.

721 *Soap Operas, Melodramas, Serials, etc.* DD: 791.457 LC: PN 1992.8F5

The value of these are mostly escapist and offer people facing a continuing flow of work decisions or series of personal problems a useful and needed chance to relax briefly in a fantasy world.

Used in this way, they may be restoring and enable a return to life's problems reinvigorated. An excessive use of this type of escapism becomes increasingly unsatisfactory and self-defeating. Conflict among values in American society are frequent themes and are interesting to analyze regardless of the ineptitude and subjectivity with which this conflict may be presented. Some useful models are presented. For instance, in some of the many detective type melodramas, the ideal way in which the police should, with fairness and justice, treat the poor and underprivileged is frequently portrayed.

722 *Comedies* DD: 791.457 LC: PN 1992.8FS

Escapism and amusement are the chief goals of these programs, yet they frequently satirize the American scene and reveal significant trends and truths. The culture gives comedians, like the court jesters in the past, special license to jest about the sacred and tabooed. Important truths in political, racial, and religious issues have been brought out in this way.

726 *News Programs and News Commentaries* DD: 971.457 LC: PN 1992.8FS, PN 4784

News programs seem to fall short of their potential more than any other type of TV presentations. They are presented too often, try to cover too much and as a consequence are superficial and biased through failing to present a many-sided view of complex problems. The viewer must constantly keep in mind the limitations of newscasting as it now exists, applying principles of propaganda analysis to everything he views and supplement this media with the more extensive reporting to be found in newspapers and weekly news magazines. Questions to ask are:

1. What pictures about the event were *not* shown?
2. Whose viewpoint about the event was *not* presented?

3. Does the commentator maintain objectivity and neutrality in what he says and in the tone of his voice?

News commentaries: it is obvious in viewing some programs that presenters are on too often, too soon after the event, or before additional information about the event has become available, even to news sleuths. News commentators with really divergent ideas about the event are rarely presented, and regular commentators share a relatively narrow range of viewpoints. The habitual viewer of these programs would do well to start a notebook in which he lists the ideological stance of each of the commentators whom he customarily views.

727 *Quiz Programs, Documentaries and Information Programs*
DD: 791.457 LC: PN 1992.8FS

Quiz programs are useful for homebound individuals who watch TV or carry on other passive activities in which there is no requirement for them to respond. Quiz programs offer the opportunity for the viewer to anticipate the answer and thus participate actively in the activity. This promotes a mental alertness and a positive interaction with mental stimuli. Once this problem-solving attitude has been achieved, it may be reapplied to other types of TV programs, such as predicting who did it in who-done-its, the points the speakers will make next in speeches, commercials, etc. This both adds zest to viewing and changes the viewer from a passive tube-drugged addict to an anticipatory, sophisticated interacting critic.

Documentaries and information programs are among the most useful of TV presentations. Through the medium of film, many places and human events may be communicated to the viewer more effectively than through any other medium. In contrast to news programs, they devote enough time to the subject to give the viewer a reasonably comprehensive coverage of the subject. Because of this slower pace, if they are biased in coverage or commentary, it becomes quickly apparent. Documentaries are especially valuable in presenting material on little known places and events, such as anthropological studies of primitive peoples.

731 Going to Circuses, Fairs, Carnivals, Amusement Parks, Rodeos, etc. DD: 791.3 LC: GV 1801-1855

There is something about the atmosphere of the circuses, carnivals, fairs, and amusement parks that makes all of us children again: fear of indigestion won't deter us from eating cotton candy and peanuts, and nobody worries about maintaining his dignity while he is riding on a roller coaster. Circuses and carnivals usually only come to an area once or twice a year; much of the fun of going to them stems from the fact that they are once-in-a-while events. Even roller coasters pall after a number of rides—even the most avid amusement park fans only visit them occasionally, lest the magic be lost.

Circuses, carnivals, and fairs provide the individual with an opportunity to participate in unusual activities while retaining his anonymity—if he wants to get excited about the prospect of hitting a target with a baseball, nobody is going to tell him he looks foolish.

Along with the festival atmosphere of circuses, carnivals, and amusement parks, fairs, especially country fairs, have the added dimension of practical purposes. Livestock, crops, and the products of farm kitchens are entered in competitions and judged, and each entrant has the opportunity to compare his work with the work of others and learn from them. Meanwhile, major manufacturers exhibit the latest in equipment, and there are many entertainment activities to thoroughly blend business and pleasure.

Carnivals, fairs, and circuses are often fund-raising events. The firemen's carnival, designed to raise money for the local fire department, is an annual event in many areas. The church fair is a particularly American institution; handmade household articles and clothing and homemade goodies are the special delights of such affairs.

The rodeo has fallen into disrepute in recent years because of the alleged cruelty to the animals involved. Critics say that techniques which may have been valid in a real-life need situation—roping and tying a steer, for example—ought not to be used for entertainment; some also claim that the "bucking broncos" are actually docile horses cruelly prodded into performing wildly.

The individual will have to decide for himself, in view of these considerations, whether he wishes to patronize rodeos. It is of course important to remember that conditions can vary greatly from one show to the next, and all ought not to be judged by the actions of what may be a minority.

Circuses, carnivals, fairs, amusement parks, rodeos, etc. are particularly suitable to group activity. They offer such a wide range of things to do and see that people of varying interests and abilities are sure to find things that will interest them. They are situations in which it is relatively easy to supervise a group, and the individual who, for example, takes a group of children to a carnival, is apt to enjoy himself quite as much as his charges do. As E.E. Cummings said, "Damn everything but the circus!"

734 *Going to Ballet and Other Dance Presentations* DD: 792.8 LC: GV 1787

Enjoyment of rhythmic movements, appreciation of meaning and emotion conveyed through the dance, these interests bring one to dance presentations.

Ballet, the most serious and disciplined of the various dance forms, is presented at its professional best by regular dance troupes and companies. Attendance at these presentations is often a glamorous affair in itself, a social event of the season. Though this is not the central attraction of the evening, still it is part of the aura that is brought to fulfillment in the ballet itself. A world is created that evening, a world which is somehow more beautiful, more mysterious, more complete than that of our everydays. That the men and women appear more than their everyday selves, that there is music and excitement and glamour in their words and demeanor, this is all fitting prelude to the world of the symbol and the abstract and the timeless reality which the dance conveys.

There is form to this fantasy however. Just as the best dancers are not the best without much work and discipline and persistence, so the heightened enjoyment of their art is not without understanding of style and technique, as well as background in music, history and literature. This is not to say that without this background the ballet cannot be enjoyed.

Forms, colors, and patterns of movement are pleasurable to most. Perhaps, though, they might find other forms of dance more to their liking. Dance expresses itself in an exciting variety, from the most primitive of rhythmic movements to carefully choreographed exercises in group coordination. People with interest in particular cultures or with strong ethnic identification might enjoy the native dances. These are often presented at the "Y" or on college campuses or at community centers. Choreography is often a central component of variety shows, talent shows, and TV specials. Tap dances, square dances, and modern dances are almost regular fare. Pleasure comes from the visual display and the rhythmical structure.

735 Going to Children's and High School Presentations of Plays, Pageants, etc. DD: 791.62 LC: PN 6120.A4-5

The anticipated lack of professional performance is often off-set by the enthusiasm of the performers and their often charming personal selves which show through the roles they are enacting. The audience not only observes the overt play but frequently a play within a play comprised of the drama of a developing personality coping with new roles. Children and youth need audiences so that player and audience become an interacting team.

Since schools are often neighborhood institutions, attending school plays and pageants is more convenient for the aged and disabled than traveling farther afield. Relatives and friends help make an enthusiastic audience.

740 Reading and Literature Appreciation Activities DD: 800 LC: PN 83

ENVIRONMENTAL FACTORS: indoor, no specific environment, modicum of space, requires little or no equipment, equipment normally at hand.

SOCIAL-PSYCHOLOGICAL FACTORS: aesthetic, utilitarian, pre-patterned, abstract, individual effort, unstructured, unsupervised, little opportunity for recognition.

Impairment Limitations

blind	S1	balance	+	*hands impaired:*	1	2
low vision	S2	seizures	+	reaching	+	+
hearing	+	*aphasia:*		handling	+	M1
speech	+	receptive	0	fingering	+	M1
retardation	0	expressive	+	feeling	+	+
memory	+	mixed	0	no hands	M1	

impaired:

stooping	+	wheel chair	+	bed patient	+
kneeling	+	semi-ambulant	+	respiratory	+
crouching	+	Class III heart	+	*Energy Expenditure in*	
crawling	+	Class IV heart	+	*METS:* 1.2	

S1 talking books and tapes
S2 large print
M1 need book holder and/or page turner

Reading can be a vital source of information and enjoyment for anyone whose contacts are limited. Information acquired through reading can give a shy individual the confidence he needs to enter into a conversation. Although reading seems a passive activity, the reader actually enters into a conversation with the author, growing in ways that are not open to the person who plants himself in front of a television set for hours of non-selective viewing. The literature of the world, accumulated over thousands of years, is varied enough to suit the taste and challenge the intellect of anyone willing to investigate his local public library.

Some of the reading and literature appreciation activities described in the following sections are available to the blind or otherwise visually impaired through the use of braille, tapes, or records (talking books).

748 *Poetry* DD: 808.81, 811 LC: PN 1010-1525

The individual who enjoys reading poetry is the kind of person who's not always in a hurry, but is willing to take time to appreciate something he likes. Poetry cannot be skimmed or read quickly; good poetry, especially, demands careful reading. Poetry is the most compact form of literature. The poet chooses each word with care, to serve a particular purpose; if the reader ignores the word, if he does not bother to ask himself "Why this word, and not another?" he is apt to lose much of the meaning of the poem.

There are many different kinds of poetry and vogues change frequently. Sometimes people refuse or are unable to recognize the value of poetry if they are not familiar and comfortable with its form; a fan of Elizabeth Barrett Browning's sonnets may not believe that the work of E.E. Cummings is "real" poetry. Most people still think of poetry in terms of rhyme and meter, lines and verses; if one has a firmly fixed notion of what poetry is, it is sometimes difficult to approach with an open mind something which does not fit that notion. Additionally, such a mystique has grown up around the reading of poetry that many people are intimidated by any poetry which they cannot comprehend immediately and easily. The process of overcoming this intimidation can often be speeded with the help of someone who is knowledgeable in the art of poetry analysis and can show that a difficult piece of poetry, if approached properly, may not be so much mysterious as it is complex and wonderful.

750 Art and Music Appreciation

ENVIRONMENTAL FACTORS: indoor, outdoor, no specific environment, modicum of space, requires little or no equipment, equipment a major factor, equipment normally at hand, equipment not necessarily at hand.

SOCIAL-PSYCHOLOGICAL FACTORS: aesthetic, pre-patterned, abstract, individual effort, structured, supervised, little opportunity for recognition.

Impairment Limitations

blind	S1	balance	+	*hands impaired:*	*1*	*2*
low vision	S1	seizures	+	reaching	+	+
hearing	S2	*aphasia:*		handling	+	+
speech	+	receptive	+	fingering	+	+
retardation	+	expressive	+	feeling	+	+
memory	+	mixed	+	no hands	+	
impaired:						
stooping	+	wheel chair	M1	bed patient	+	
kneeling	+	semi-ambulant	M1	respiratory	+	
crouching	+	Class III heart	+	*Energy Expenditure in*		
crawling	+	Class IV heart	0	*METS:* 1.2-3.2		

S1 except art gallery and museums
S2 except lectures and music
M1 check on whether ramps or elevators give access to buildings, check availability of toilet facilities

752 Group Listening and/or Discussion of Records, Tapes, Programs, etc. DD: 789.91 LC: LB 1044.4, 1044.3

Listening to music in groups may be very informal and spontaneous or somewhat planned as get-togethers with family or friends. Visitors may be asked to bring some of their own records or tapes for more variety, or records may be borrowed from public libraries. The purpose may be simply to share the music or to promote other activities such as singing, playing instruments, dancing or partying. Persons may want to gather for specific musical programs on radio or television for any of the above reasons or for educational value.

Groups may also gather to listen in order to learn about various kinds of music forms. Listening to the recording of an opera or a symphony before attending a live performance may facilitate a more complete understanding and appreciation of the performance. Groups may gather at a member's home or find some central location, perhaps a listening room at a local library, church or agency.

A vital area of music appreciation, that of individual interpretations and attitudes, can be covered in group discussions. In a heterogeneous group, individuals can learn from one another and develop their own attitudes and tastes. Discussing ideas and feelings about music may concretize vague impressions and develop fluency of expressions. Musicians among the group might be encouraged to add to discussions with their knowledge of musical skills and structure or by playing and/or singing. Individuals can make this a regular activity by enrolling in music appreciation courses or joining music study clubs or listening groups, if accessible in the community.

755 Attending Lectures and/or Taking Courses on Music DD: 781 LC: MT

This type of activity may be pursued by the musician who wishes to intensify and complement his active musical work (e.g., composer, director, singer, instrumentalist), or it may be sought by one whose interest in music is more abstract—theory, development, history of music. The courses for either may be the same. They are offered by colleges and universities, by conservatories and other schools of music, and sometimes even by secondary schools. The courses may deal with the highly rigorous and regulated principles of classical music, the improvisations of jazz and non-Western music, or the simpler rhythms and melodies of popular music.

The non-musician who treasures his musical sense will value these contacts with the musical world. TV broadcasts (e.g., Leonard Bernstein's Young People's Concerts) and library resources (published lectures and other works on music) have the advantages of formal lectures and courses without the physical and financial demands.

757 *Going to Museums and Public Art Galleries* DD: 708, 726.7 LC: AM, N 400-490

Museums and public galleries cater to the wide variety of public tastes in art, although some specialize, collecting and showing one type of art. Admission is usually free; visitors have complete freedom to look at as many or as few works as desired or can go on tours. Since mind and feelings, which are utilized in looking at works of art, are faculties which tire easily, it is recommended that individuals look at relatively few works of art in each visit. Persons who spend only three to four seconds on each work do not really see; they miss the artistic experience and are not engaging in an art appreciation activity.

Much can be learned by this activity, e.g., ability to recognize artist's styles and famous works. Desire to learn more about art or even to develop one's own talents might be another by-product.

This activity, although not physically strenuous, requires a good deal of standing and walking around; persons who tire very easily can plan to sit down at intervals. Conditions of museums and galleries should be known for persons who might have difficulty entering and leaving and/or climbing stairs.

760 *Traveling*

ENVIRONMENTAL FACTORS: outdoor, no specific environment, unlimited space, requires little or no equipment, equipment normally at hand.

SOCIAL-PSYCHOLOGICAL FACTORS: aesthetic, creative, pre-patterned, concrete, group effort, individual effort, structured, unstructured, supervised, unsupervised, opportunity for recognition, little opportunity for recognition.

Impairment Limitations

blind	M1	balance	M2	*hands impaired:*	1	2
low vision	+	seizures	M2	reaching	+	+
hearing	+	*aphasia:*		handling	+	+
speech	+	receptive	M2	fingering	+	+
retardation	M2	expressive	M2	feeling	+	+
memory	M2	mixed	M2	no hands	+	

impaired:

stooping	+	wheel chair	M3	bed patient	0
kneeling	+	semi-ambulant	+	respiratory	+
crouching	+	Class III heart	+	*Energy Expenditure in*	
crawling	+	Class IV heart	0	*METS:* 1.2-4.5	

M1 need sighted companion
M2 need companion for guidance and protection
M3 need folding wheelchair for car

762 *Trips to Visit Friends, Relatives* DD: 910.2-.4 LC: G 149-157, G 200-306

Visits to friends and relatives are very important to maintain close social ties. In a society where there is frequent moving about in search of jobs, education, training or taking better jobs, the continuation of long-term friendships and contacts with relatives becomes increasingly important for a sense of belonging. Frequent visiting improves the relationships, which can also be improved by planning on how the relationship can best be augmented. This may include planning to avoid topics on which there is disagreement or planning to inquire about the things about which the other person may be very knowledgeable but does not voice in ordinary conversation. For instance, older relatives frequently have fascinating stories of their childhood experiences. Some relationships thrive on a non-verbal basis such as playing chess or checkers.

763 *Trips to enjoy Seasonal Scenery* DD: 910.2-.4 LC: G 149-157, G 200-306

These trips might be local or long-distance ones made to see unusual sights, usually made by car. Local sights might be the dogwood, bluebonnet or azalea trails and garden tours, or the acres of apple blossoms or large pansy beds near towns. One might travel some distance in order to see the cherry blossoms in Washington, D.C., or the autumn foliage or snow-covered hills of northern climates. The enjoyment of these trips may be enhanced by photographing, sketching or painting scenes or by classifying and collecting botanical specimens.

770 *Religious Activities* DD: 291.7 LC: BX

ENVIRONMENTAL FACTORS: indoor, no specific environment, modicum of space, requires little or no equipment, equipment normally at hand.

SOCIAL-PSYCHOLOGICAL FACTORS: aesthetic, pre-patterned, abstract, group effort, individual effort, structured, supervised, opportunity for recognition.

Impairment Limitations

blind	M1	balance	+	*hands impaired:*	*1*	*2*
low vision	+	seizures	+	reaching	+	+
hearing	+	*aphasia:*		handling	+	+
speech	+	receptive	+	fingering	+	+
retardation	+	expressive	+	feeling	+	+
memory	+	mixed	+	no hands	+	
impaired:						
stooping	+	wheel chair	M2	bed patient	S2	
kneeling	+	semi-ambulant	M2	respiratory	+	
crouching	+	Class III heart	+	*Energy Expenditure in*		
crawling	+	Class IV heart	S1	*METS:* 1.2-3.2		

M1 may need sighted companion
M2 check on whether ramps or elevators give access to church buildings
    and availability of toilet facilities
S1 limited to religious activities carried on at home

Religious activities are manifestations of a person's most subjective experience. The religious experience is personal, individual, and at the same time carried on within a social context. The values one affirms as a result of his religious experience give a unity to his personal life and form the basis for social relationships. Religious affiliation provides a context within which one establishes his personal identity. Religious orientation may foster a sense of personal growth and a sense of community.

Whether or not one gives even tacit acceptance to religious behavior as an authentic expression of human experience, one can hardly deny it is a powerful influence, especially in altering or fostering behavioral characteristics. A powerful religious experience will often be cited as the turning point in a person's life. This might seem the ideal tool with which to sublimate or redirect destructive or ineffective social traits, but its very strength is its weakness. The religious experience is intensely personal, very subjective and may easily incorporate other than religious influences into its expression. Outside interference into an established religious system is a tricky business and usually not a very profitable one. Even those to whom the authority is ordained (e.g., Catholic priests, who have enjoyed this kind of deference more than most other ministers of faith) cannot always break through the shield of religious defences. Religion may be used as the justification for all manner of selfish and nonreligious acts, but only those who wish to listen will hear of their failings.

It should be recognized that participation in religious activities gives one a sense of fellowship, belonging, identity, personal worth and transcendence of self. The activities appeal to emotional, spiritual, and intellectual dimensions of a person's life. One person's form of participation may not be another's.

778 Participation in Pilgrimages and Retreats DD: 291.38 LC: BV 5068, BX 2375

These are special occasions of religious activity. Pilgrimages are usually to a particular location which represents some special person or event. Some pilgrimages incorporate voluntary inflictions of physical hardships as well as rejoicing. Participation in a pilgrimage presupposes a certain kind of devotion not common to all. Retreats are more widely practiced. They are designed to give one "time out" to evaluate and readjust religious conceptions and practices, especially in regard to everyday life. Retreats may be directed towards a particular group, e.g., engaged couples, high school seniors, etc. They work best when voluntarily entered into. Forced retreats, especially among teen-agers, develop into a game of who can best frustrate the purpose.

780 Self-development Activities

Self development activities: includes skill improvement courses such as cooking, woodworking, etc.

ENVIRONMENTAL FACTORS: indoor, outdoor, no specific environment, specialized environment and/or climate, modicum of space, unlimited space, requires little or no equipment, equipment a major factor, equipment normally at hand, equipment not necessarily at hand.

SOCIAL-PSYCHOLOGICAL FACTORS: aesthetic, utilitarian, creative, pre-patterned, concrete, group effort, individual effort, structured, unstructured, supervised, unsupervised, opportunity for recognition, little opportunity for recognition.

Impairment Limitations

blind	S1	balance	S5	*hands impaired:*	1	2
low vision	S2	seizures	S5	reaching	+	M1
hearing	+	*aphasia:*		handling	+	M1
speech	+	receptive	S3	fingering	+	M1
retardation	S3	expressive	+	feeling	M2	M2
memory	S4	mixed	S3	no hands	M1	

impaired:

stooping	M3	wheel chair	S6	bed patient	S7, S8
kneeling	M3	semi-ambulant	S6	respiratory	S7
crouching	M3	Class III heart	S7	*Energy Expenditure in*	
crawling	M3	Class IV heart	S7, S8	*METS:* 1.2-8	

M1 use vise, jigs, and fixtures in cooking, woodworking
M2 protect against burns, cuts and bruises in cooking, woodworking, etc.
M3 avoid lower extremity exercises unless therapeutically prescribed
S1 use tapes, talking books, braille
S2 everything but speed reading

S3   avoid demanding intellectual activities
S4   take more notes or record on tape
S5   avoid hazardous activities in cooking, woodworking, etc.
S6   check on whether ramps or elevators give access to buildings and avail-
ability of toilet facilities
S7   avoid strenuous exercise
S8   can carry on academic activities at home

781 *Figure Control, Exercises, Yoga, etc.* DD: 646.75 LC: GV 461-547, RM 721

Advocates of physical fitness programs are forever repeating how important is one's physical condition to one's mental health. "Healthy mind in a healthy body" is the resounding cry and it is echoed with equal fervor by advocates of programs on improving mental health. Thus hounded from all sides, what's a physical misfit to do? Only the staunchest dare sit back and, with a broad smile, pop yet another chocolate into his mouth. His more guilt-ridden partners-in-crime will engage meanwhile in all manner of weight-reducing activities: enrollment in the "Y" will undergo a phenomenal increase, parks and side roads will be flooded with joggers and the countryside will resound with anguished cries resulting from stiff muscles and sore joints.

In time, the result may be a few more listed among the ranks of the physically fit. They will be reaping the mental benefits of their new top-shape condition, eating less, sleeping better, working and playing longer. They will swell the ranks of the militant health-mongers, exhorting one and all to "shape up," and holding aloft their banner "A thinner tomorrow is a better tomorrow."

In the meantime, the less persevering, having succumbed to their former habits, have left the sauna room at the gym and have rejoined their friend around a box of chocolates. Happiness is where you find it.

782 *Charm and Poise Courses* DD: 646.72-.73 LC: BJ 1609-1610

Charm and poise courses are based on Hans Christian Anderson's premise that ugly ducklings can be transformed into lovely, graceful swans. Real life, however, does not always attain to fairy-tale heights. Some of the ducklings, despite the most heroic efforts, will never reach swandom. However, all is not lost. Charm and poise courses can make ugly ducklings into rather attractive ducklings, or at least, well, ducklings. The best a course could offer would be to teach the duckling the basics of how to make the most of herself—to disguise flaws and play up good features, and thus improve her mental conception of herself, which is probably the single most important factor in appearance. She might then be a happier duckling. So who needs more swans??

784 *Vocabulary Development* DD: 428.2 LC: P 305

A diverse vocabulary is normally developed through the years by extensive reading of varied materials and listening to and conversing with individuals with wide-range vocabularies. This includes attending lectures, plays and poetry readings. More specific attempts to improve vocabularies may be made through learning lists of new words and using a thesaurus to develop greater variety and precision in word usage. Vocabulary development is a two-edged sword; while it can lead to better communication, it can also lead to a pretentious artificiality in which complicated words are used for effect rather than for precision. The most sophisticated vocabulary development is that in which the speaker uses the array of words best suited to the particular individual or audience he is addressing at the time. If the listener is used to four letter words, use four letter words if you wish to be understood.

790 *Miscellaneous Education, Cultural and Entertainment Activities*

Miscellaneous education, cultural and entertainment activities: including debating, public speaking, dining out and night club going.

ENVIRONMENTAL FACTORS: indoor, outdoor, no specific environment specialized environment and/or climate, modicum of space, requires little or no equipment, equipment a major factor, equipment normally at hand, equipment not necessarily at hand.

SOCIAL-PSYCHOLOGICAL FACTORS: aesthetic, utilitarian, creative, pre-patterned, concrete, group effort, individual effort, structured, unstructured, supervised, unsupervised, opportunity for recognition, little opportunity for recognition.

Impairment Limitations

					hands impaired:	1	2
blind	M1		balance	M3	*hands impaired:*	1	2
low vision	+		seizures	M4	reaching	+	+
hearing	S1		*aphasia:*		handling	+	M5
speech	S1		receptive	S1	fingering	+	M5
retardation	S1		expressive	S1	feeling	+	+
memory	S1,	M2	mixed	S1	no hands	M5	

impaired:

stooping	+	wheel chair	M6	bed patient	0	
kneeling	+	semi-ambulant	M6	respiratory	+	
crouching	+	Class III heart	+	*Energy Expenditure in*		
crawling	+	Class IV heart	0	*METS:* 1.2-3.2		

M1 may need sighted companion
M2 record names of guests for ready reference
M3 problem in drinking establishments of being labeled as tipsy or drunk
M4 avoid drinking alcohol
M5 may need companion to assist in feeding
M6 check accessibility to restaurants, etc., by ramps or elevators and accessibility of suitable toilet facilities
S1 except debate, public speaking, forensics

791 *Informal Entertaining* DD: 791, 395, 642.41 LC: GV 1470-1561, TX 731-9

Informal entertaining performs a very important function in improving interpersonal relations. Although the charm of informal entertaining is in its spontaneity, careful preplanning of some details such as where chairs are placed and when food is served may make the difference between fun and boredom. The participants also have roles to play to add to the success of the party. These include: making strangers feel comfortable, being a good listener to the recitation of the achievements or problems of other participants, and showing the proper appreciation for the effort the hostess or host has put forth to arrange the get-together.

792 Formal Entertaining DD: 642.4, 395.3, 791 LC: TX 851-885,
BJ 2021-2038

Formal entertaining usually involves more structuring of the
situation with respect to time, dress, timing, who's invited and
the probability of setting up a chain of reciprocal engagements.
Formal entertaining serves a useful social function in getting together individuals or groups who would not interact as favorably
in either a business/professional meeting or at an informal gather-
ing. In contrast to informal entertaining, the hostess or host is
expected to make elaborate preparations and the guests have
more explicit obligations in terms of accepting or rejecting the
invitation, dress, arriving on time and providing reciprocal benefits. Formal entertaining usually requires more structured role
playing and role maintaining than is to be found in informal
entertaining and inferences about this are suggested by the formality of introductions and by titles used.

800 Volunteer Activities

This section on Volunteer Activities requires some extensive
explanation. In general, the job tasks performed in volunteer
activities are similar to those performed by paid workers, and the
reader is referred to the Dictionary of Occupational Titles for
information on the job tasks involved. The rules, regulations,
hours of work, and the social situation under which the work
is carried on tends to be different. Since the volunteer receives no
pay, it is assumed that intrinsic rewards must be available to
assure his motivation. That it is intrinsically meaningful and
satisfying to a volunteer to help either an individual or an organization which he believes is worthy of support is a value assumption which we have made.

In general, volunteers with occupational experience at the
skilled level or above will have most to contribute as consultants,
teachers, tutors, trainers, supervisors and advisers to young people
who are considering entering the occupation. In some volunteer
activities, however, the volunteer performs the actual job much
as those who are paid for the work. As an example, a Red Cross
volunteer driver transports patients in an automobile just as

does a taxi driver, although the rules, regulations, hours of work and the social situation are different. In addition to describing what volunteers have traditionally done in the past, we have also suggested other possibilities. Some of these involve organizing and training people in the use of industrial processes and expensive equipment. This makes an assumption with which the reader may or may not agree—that it is desirable to help new small economic units such as cooperatives, communes, and small businesses operated by the disadvantaged, including the handicapped and minority group members, get started. This is based on the postulate that small businesses make for a more healthy economy and a more stable society. An additional value assumption is made that a racially integrated society is desirable.

810 Professional, Technical and Managerial Activities

Professional, technical and managerial activities: including drafting and sports umpiring.

ENVIRONMENTAL FACTORS: indoor, no specific environment, modicum of space, requires little or no equipment, equipment normally at hand.

SOCIAL-PSYCHOLOGICAL FACTORS: utilitarian, creative, pre-patterned, abstract, concrete, individual effort, structured, supervised, opportunity for recognition.

Impairment Limitations

blind	S1	balance	+	*hands impaired:*	1	2
low vision	S1	seizures	+	reaching	+	S1
hearing	S2	*aphasia:*		handling	+	S1
speech	S2	receptive	0	fingering	+	S1
retardation	0	expressive	0	feeling	+	S1
memory	0	mixed	0	no hands	S1	

impaired:

stooping	+	wheel chair	+	bed patient	0
kneeling	+	semi-ambulant	+	respiratory	+
crouching	+	Class III heart	+	*Energy Expenditure in*
crawling	+	Class IV heart	0	*METS:* 1.4-3.5

S1 exclude drafting, umpiring
S2 exclude umpiring

810 Professional, Technical and Managerial Activities

At times, when these activities are carried on in a volunteer capacity, it is difficult to differentiate them from paid work situations. For instance, some corporations loan executives to work on United Appeal Campaigns. Other corporations encourage their executives to be active in community organizations, which frequently involves carrying on some of the activities on company time.

When performed on a volunteer basis, the teaching, tutoring, consulting, and advising of young people who are considering entering the professional aspects of the activities tend to be stressed. Usually volunteer services offered in these categories are offered by retired professionals.

811 Mathematics, Physical and Biological Sciences

Mathematics, physical and biological sciences: e.g., programmers, chemists, horticulturists, etc. DD: 510, 530, 574. LC: Q 181.

Volunteers with these competences can be useful in the guidance of math, physics, biology, chemistry and garden clubs. They also can be of help in botanical gardens, zoos, museums, arboretums, and planetariums. Psychologists can help with individual problems and as group leaders and consultants.

812 Social Sciences

Social Sciences: e.g., economists, historians, etc. DD: 300, 330. LC: HM 131.

Historians are useful as participants and advisers in local history and genealogy research. Local newspapers are an excellent source of local historical information. Historians can supervise other volunteers in collecting, organizing and reporting on specialized local historical developments in the field of industry, education, the arts, music, or other topics of interest. Developing the genealogy of long established families for which this has not been done is also of interest.

Political scientists can work in political parties, help run political campaigns, work in and advise such groups as the League of Women Voters and Common Cause. Sociologists can help plan organizational structures and analyze organizational functioning, do research and advise on research on social problems.

Anthropologists can lead and advise anthropology and archeology clubs and conduct archeological searches in local areas.

820 Clerical and Sales Activities

ENVIRONMENTAL FACTORS: indoor, no specific environment, modicum of space, equipment a major factor, equipment normally at hand.

SOCIAL-PSYCHOLOGICAL FACTORS: utilitarian, pre-patterned, concrete, individual effort, structured, supervised, little opportunity for recognition.

Impairment Limitations

					hands impaired:	1	2
blind	S1	balance	+		reaching	S3	S3
low vision	S1	seizures	+		handling	S3	S3
hearing	S2	*aphasia:*			fingering	S3	S3
speech	S2	receptive	0		feeling	+	S3
retardation	0	expressive	0		no hands	S3	
memory	0	mixed	0				

impaired:						
stooping	+	wheel chair	+	bed patient	S4	
kneeling	+	semi-ambulant	+	respiratory	+	
crouching	+	Class III heart	+	*Energy Expenditure in*		
crawling	+	Class IV heart	0	*METS:* 1.4-3		

S1 typing, sales
S2 exclude telephone operator, stenographer, receptionist, sales
S3 exclude stenography, typing, filing
S4 can do telephone canvassing

821 Stenography, Typing, Filing, and Related Activities DD: 651.3743, 652.3, 651.5 LC: HF 5436-5746, Z 53, Z 56, Z 49-50, HF 5547

A great deal of the typing for political and special causes groups is done by volunteers, many of them homemakers with prior paid clerical experience. This provides the satisfaction of contributing to a cause of meaningful social significance. When these clerical workers get together in a common meeting place, to the satisfaction of completing the work is added the pleasures of social companionship. The volunteer job of secretary is found in nearly every avocational organization.

824 Information and Message Distribution Activities, e.g., messengers, telephone operators, etc. DD: 651.374 LC: TK 6163-T, HE

There has been a recent rapid expansion of this kind of volunteer in the development of underground switchboard activities. Many problems have arisen which are not resolved with respect to the professional level responsibilities thrust upon these telephone information answering services. It is likely that there will be extensive training programs developed for people entering this kind of volunteer work in the future. A telephone network service for elderly and disabled people to provide them with both protection and companionship is a greatly needed volunteer service.

825 Salesmen Services DD: 658.85 LC: HF 5438-9

There is a continuing demand for volunteer salesmen as placement officers to place disadvantaged individuals. Retired people who have had managerial positions can be particularly effective at this because of their contacts in the business world. Real estate salesmen can be of help in sponsoring integrated housing. Stock and bond salesmen can aid cooperatives, communes and small businesses operated by the handicapped and minority group members raise capital for starting or expanding their businesses.

830 Service Activities

ENVIRONMENTAL FACTORS: indoor, outdoor, no specific environment, modicum of space, requires little or no equipment, equipment normally at hand.

SOCIAL-PSYCHOLOGICAL FACTORS: utilitarian, pre-patterned, concrete, individual effort, structured, supervised, little opportunity for recognition.

Impairment Limitations

blind	0	balance	S1	*hands impaired:*	1	2	
low vision	+	seizures	S1	reaching	S2	S2	
hearing	S1	*aphasia:*		handling	S2	S2	
speech	+	receptive	0	fingering	S2	S2	
retardation	+	expressive	S1	feeling	M1	M1	
memory	S1	mixed	0	no hands	S3		

impaired:

stooping	+	wheel chair	0	bed patient	0
kneeling	+	semi-ambulant	0	respiratory	+
crouching	+	Class III heart	+	*Energy Expenditure in*	
crawling	+	Class IV heart	0	*METS:* 1.2-4.5	

M1 avoid contact with hot stove and hot containers in cooking
S1 exclude waiters, watchmen, guards
S2 exclude barbering, janitors, cooks, guards
S3 could be watchman, barker, usher

831 Domestic Service Activities, e.g., baby sitting, yardmen, etc.
DD: 649.10248, 647.3 LC: RJ 61, RJ 101, SB 451-466, HQ 769-780

Volunteer baby sitting is an extremely valuable service which many people who are limited in their other skills can do. This is particularly important in freeing mothers to vote, to secure medical services for themselves or for their children, to shop, and to carry out other essential errands.

Volunteer sitters are greatly needed for elderly disabled couples where, as in some stroke cases, the patient needs constant supervision, and the spouse can hardly ever get out of the house to go shopping.

Volunteer sitters receive not only the satisfaction of helping but the fun of watching the fascinating drama of children at play.

Volunteers who sit with the elderly disabled frequently are rewarded with the many interesting stories elderly people have to tell about past experiences and observations.

Various innovative projects which have been tried are "foster grandparents" who take an interest in children in institutions, locating day care centers for children in nursing homes and having mentally retarded children cared for by mentally ill women patients.

There is an unlimited need for yardmen to clean up vacant lots, plant flowers, grass and shrubs on unused public lands, etc. The many beautiful public parks in Canadian cities are models which the United States might well emulate.

To replace the ugly chaos of American cities with the beauty of growing things is for many an aesthetically satisfying volunteer activity.

833 Lodging and Related Service Activities, e.g., bellmen, housing exchange students, etc. DD: 728.7, 647.2 LC: HD 7288, HD 4801-4942

The growth of various kinds of foster homes and halfway houses to some extent replaces the extended kinship family in offering living facilities outside the nucleus of a family. The influence of the volunteer in providing much needed love, affection, supervision and protection far exceeds the mere providing of a place to stay.

Housing exchange students may be as much of a learning experience for the hostess or host as for the student.

834 Barbering, Cosmetology and Related Service Activities DD: 646.72 LC: TT 950-979

A much more effective presentation of self in every day life is possible with the improved physical appearance attributable to barbering and cosmetology. Volunteer instructors in cosmetology have been effectively used in work adjustment programs as part of the orientation to work training offered.

The self image of long term mental patients, particularly, may be improved through helping them to improve their appearance.

837 Protective Service Activities, e.g., crossing watchmen, guards, etc. DD: 363.2-.3 LC: HV 8290

There is an almost unlimited need for volunteer school crossing guards. With increased violence and disorderly conduct in inner city schools, volunteer guards could be most useful, probably under some other name, such as playground attendant. Volunteer firemen are an established institution in suburban and rural areas. There are also opportunities in volunteer auxiliary police forces although this has the social hazards of possible violation of civil liberties. Assigning these auxiliary police to first aid squads may be a way out of this dilemma.

840 Farming, Fishery and Forestry Activities

ENVIRONMENTAL FACTORS: outdoor, specialized environment and/or climate, unlimited space, equipment a major factor, equipment not necessarily at hand.

SOCIAL-PSYCHOLOGICAL FACTORS: utilitarian, pre-patterned, concrete, group effort, individual effort, structured, supervised, opportunity for recognition.

Impairment Limitations

				hands impaired:	1	2
blind	0	balance	M1			
low vision	S1	seizures	M1	reaching	+	0
hearing	+	*aphasia:*		handling	+	0
speech	+	receptive	S1	fingering	+	0
retardation	+	expressive	S1	feeling	M2	M2
memory	M1	mixed	S1	no hands	0	

impaired:

stooping	M3	wheel chair	0	bed patient	0
kneeling	M3	semi-ambulant	0	respiratory	+
crouching	M3	Class III heart	0	*Energy Expenditure in*	
crawling	+	Class IV heart	0	*METS:* 3.2-5.6	

M1 need companion for safety
M2 avoid cuts from sharp instruments, scratches from thorns, etc.
M3 use tools which make it unnecessary to carry out these physical activities
S1 can do farming, forestry, not hunting

841 Plant Farming Activities DD: 635 LC: S-SB 51

Many growers of vegetable gardens find themselves giving away a large part of their extra produce to friends, neighbors and relatives to the point where it becomes a kind of volunteer activity. If every vegetable gardener would grow a little extra and undertake to supply the needs of one family on welfare the dire poverty in which welfare families now live could be lessened.

844 Forestry Activities, e.g., ecology DD: 581.54, 581.5222-.5223 LC: SD

Boy Scouts and 4-H Clubs have traditionally undertaken extensive volunteer work in planting evergreen seedlings. With the recent increased interest in ecology it is hoped that many other groups and individuals will undertake this volunteer work.

There are many parcels of public lands not only in rural but in suburban and even metropolitan areas on which trees could be planted if the volunteers to do it were available.

880 Structural Work Activities

ENVIRONMENTAL FACTORS: indoor, outdoor, no specific environment, modicum of space, equipment a major factor, equipment not necessarily at hand.

SOCIAL-PSYCHOLOGICAL FACTORS: utilitarian, pre-patterned, concrete, group effort, individual effort, structured, supervised, opportunity for recognition.

Impairment Limitations

blind	0	balance	M1	*hands impaired:*	1	2
low vision	0	seizures	M1	reaching	+	M2
hearing	+	*aphasia:*		handling	+	M2
speech	+	receptive	+	fingering	+	M2
retardation	+	expressive	+	feeling	+	M3
memory	+	mixed	+	no hands	M2	

impaired:					
stooping	S1	wheel chair	S1	bed patient	0
kneeling	S1	semi-ambulant	S1	respiratory	M4
crouching	S1	Class III heart	M4	*Energy Expenditure in*	
crawling	S1	Class IV heart	0	*METS:* 2.0-10.5	

M1 avoid high places, moving machinery
M2 use reachers, vises
M3 avoid sharp objects, heat
M4 light work, slow pace, short time
S1   work at waist height or above

880 Structural Work Activities LC: T 355, TG 260

Volunteers in structural work activities have been traditional since the barn raising parties of pioneer days. Many churches have been built entirely with volunteer labor. Currently, with the complicated building codes and legalized occupational monopolies in urban areas, a considerable amount of volunteer structural work must be limited to rural areas.

884 Painting, Plastering, Cementing, Waterproofing and Related Activities DD: 667.6, 693.6 LC: TT 300-380, TH 8120-8137, TH 1461-1501

There is an unlimited amount of this type of repair work to be done for nonprofit organizations and for elderly and disabled people who are not able to do it for themselves. This is particularly suitable for volunteers who like to help people in a personal way but do not enjoy social interaction with people. Interior painting has unique opportunities for handicapped volunteers. Much of it can be done with one hand, and there is an aesthetic satisfaction to be gained from the color schemes selected and a high sense of achievement for the amount of money and work invested.

890 Miscellaneous Volunteer Activities

ENVIRONMENTAL FACTORS: indoor, outdoor, no specific environment, specialized environment and/or climate, modicum of space, unlimited space, equipment a major factor, equipment normally at hand.

SOCIAL-PSYCHOLOGICAL FACTORS: utilitarian, pre-patterned, concrete, group effort, individual effort, structured, supervised, opportunity for recognition.

Impairment Limitations

blind	0	balance	S1	*hands impaired:*	1	2
low vision	0	seizures	S1	reaching	+	S2
hearing	+	*aphasia:*		handling	+	S2
speech	+	receptive	0	fingering	+	S2
retardation	0	expressive	0	feeling	+	+
memory	0	mixed	0	no hands	S2	
impaired:						
stooping	+	wheel chair	S1	bed patient	0	
kneeling	+	semi-ambulant	S1	respiratory	+	
crouching	+	Class III heart	+	*Energy Expenditure in*		
crawling	+	Class IV heart	0	*METS:* 1.8-6		

S1 can do graphic work; avoid driving, motor freight activities
S2 avoid driving, motor freight activities

892 *Transportation Activities, n.e.c.* DD: 385-388 LC: HE

Volunteer drivers are greatly in demand to transport clients
and patients in their own cars or agency cars. The Red Cross has
been instrumental in organizing this service, but there never
seems to be enough of it to go around.

898 *Activities in Graphics Work* DD: 760 LC: NC

Because of the widespread amateur interest in art, art work
professionals are frequently needed as instructors in art classes.
Darkroom specialists are helpful instructors in camera courses and
camera clubs. Bookbinders may enjoy working on limited editions
of volumes on local history and genealogy.

900 *Organizational Activities*

The social setting within which an activity is carried on is
structured partly by the nature of the activity and partly by external events. For many participants, the social setting is more
important than the nature of the activity itself. The hackneyed
example is that of the insurance salesman who plays golf at the
"right" golf club in order to meet affluent business executives.
The second overworked example is that of the use of coed activities as a way to meet a potential marriage partner.

The nature of the activity influences the social setting in a
number of ways. For instance, extremely vigorous activities narrow the age range of those who can participate. In some cases,
there are minimum age limits to obtain a license to participate
in the activity, such as in automobile driving. These reduce the
generation gap, with closer interpersonal relationships as a result.

Events which require the participants to travel somewhere and
stay overnight lead to closer interpersonal relationships, as they
get to know each other in roles other than as activity participants.
Thus the sparkling conversationalist in a social evening at the
ski lodge has an opportunity to offset a perhaps bungling performance on the bunny hill.

Shared danger brings people closer together and one would expect to find a close camaraderie among parachute jumpers and auto racers as a result. Where the participant's safety depends upon his teammates, the bonding effect of danger is likely to be multiplied, and one would anticipate mountain climbing teams to have especially close interpersonal relationships.

All activities develop a folklore known only to the initiated and one which constitutes a continuing source of conversation. Activities with regularly scheduled exciting events, particularly races, constantly add to the fund of folklore so that stale conversation is continually recycled.

Organized activities require "organization men" (and women) to keep them going and status may be gained in any of the ubiquitous president, vice-president, secretary and treasurer's positions. As a holder of one of these positions, the participant may be assured of being an accepted member of the in-group even though his performance as a participant of the activity may be inferior.

All clubs, of course, serve the function of bringing together people with similar interests.

915 Self-Defense, e.g., boxing, wrestling, karate, fencing DD: 796.78153, 796.83, 796.86, 796.812 LC: U 860-863, GV 476, GV 1195, GV 1115-1141

Combat sports such as wrestling, karate and fencing have been incorporated into many recreational programs; however, boxing as a competitive sport for youth has been generally discouraged. Wrestling and fencing programs are being carried on in high schools, recreation departments, church athletic programs and YMCA and boys' club organizations. The YWCA and some school physical education programs include fencing in the activities for girls. It should be noted that the introduction of these types of sports into activity programs requires careful orientation of the participants and constant supervision of regular practice sessions until the sport is learned.

The interpersonal relationships in boxing, wrestling and judo are distinctive in that participants more or less continuously inflict pain on their opponents. This requires participants to develop a strong control over anger normally felt toward a source which inflicts pain. Special emotional control is required to pursue the tactics of the sport most likely to win the match rather than opting for a tactic which inflicts the most pain as a reprisal.

Being on the receiving end of the pain inflicted in these sports requires special training in maintaining social composure and an appropriate presentation of self while withstanding a degree of pain which might elicit tears and whimpering in the untrained. Males brought up in low income and disadvantaged areas where street fighting is commonplace are apt to have had much more intensive and appropriate training for this role.

922 Art Clubs e.g., painting, sculpture, photography, etc. DD: 730, 750, 770 LC: TR, ND, NB

In these clubs the activity itself is usually solitary and the interpersonal relationships involved are adjunctive to the activity itself. The interchange with other club members is focused on having an audience to whom to show off one's work, getting help on problems, sharing ideas for new subject matter and techniques, and sharing equipment, darkroom and model costs.

Exchanging ideas with others is frequently necessary to incite and increase creativity; the club also serves this purpose. Sharing enthusiasm over an art product requires a certain kind of positive empathy which only the artistically inclined person is likely to have. For example, nearly everyone responds emotionally to the dramatic impact of any kind of a race but only those specially prepared will respond to a particular painting or sculpture.

925 Card Game Clubs, e.g., bridge, poker, sheepshead, etc. DD: 795.4 LC: GV 1233-1299

Card clubs often exist as part of a larger formal or informal organization, such as a church or a secretarial pool.

Specific games seem to have become primarily associated with specific social groups. Thus, bridge tends to be comprised of married couples for evening games and women groups for afternoon games. A rather unique form of communication between partners is required in bridge in which the partner is expected to understand what his partner can and expects to do through his ritualized statements. Ineptness in either sending or receiving these communications in required style tends to trigger the partner's wrath. In husband-wife teams, there is likely to be a great deal of displacement of antagonisms in other role performances due to the game performance.

Poker is primarily a man's game, frequently played compulsively late into the night. Money stakes are frequently higher than in other games and appropriate emotional control is required to sustain relatively heavy financial losses without destroying friendships. In this respect it is similar to body contact sports. The game mimics the chief ingredients of many buying and selling jobs in which the key to success is bluffing the opponent into believing that the participant is in a stronger position than he really is. This involves maintaining a special kind of presentation of self including appropriate facial expressions and tone of voice.

928 Craft Clubs, e.g., cooking, sewing, gardening, etc. DD: 641.5-.8, 646, 647.3 LC: TX 645-840, SB 451-466, TT 700-715

Craft clubs like art clubs are organized around the pursuit of activities which result in a finished product. However, some craft products like cooked meals are perishable. This has implications for craft clubs as it may determine how frequently and when meetings are held. Certain species of flowers bloom only at certain times of the year and meetings of these kinds of clubs may be in accord with this.

Mutual sharing products of cookery crafts is perhaps a more demanding experience in interpersonal relationships than the aesthetic sharing in art clubs. The figurative interpretation of the phrase "I can't stomach that" is less painful than is the literal.

As in art clubs, activities are primarily carried on as individual projects. Sewing is somewhat unique in that, except when new and complicated stitches are being learned, sewers are able to converse while sewing. Thus sewing clubs may be concurrently conversational clubs.

The 4-H clubs and Future Farmers of America have long been

active in organizing craft clubs for the display of their products at state and county fairs.

930 *Political Groups*

ENVIRONMENTAL FACTORS: indoor, outdoor, no specific environment, modicum of space, requires little or no equipment, equipment normally at hand.

SOCIAL-PSYCHOLOGICAL FACTORS: aesthetic, utilitarian, creative, pre-patterned, abstract, concrete, group effort, individual effort, structured, supervised, opportunity for recognition.

Impairment Limitations

blind	+	balance	+	*hands impaired:*	*1*	*2*
low vision	+	seizures	+	reaching	+	+
hearing	S1	*aphasia:*		handling	+	+
speech	S2	receptive	S3	fingering	+	+
retardation	S3	expressive	S3	feeling	+	+
memory	S3	mixed	S3	no hands	+	

impaired:

stooping	+	wheel chair	M1	bed patient	S4
kneeling	+	semi-ambulant	M1	respiratory	+
crouching	+	Class III heart	+	*Energy Expenditure in*	
crawling	+	Class IV heart	S4	*METS:* 1.2-4.4	

M1 check access to buildings via ramps and elevators and suitability of toilet facilities
S1 read instructions and speeches rather than listen to them
S2 can perform all activities except speaking to people
S3 can stuff envelopes, put on car tops, bumper stickers
S4 can dictate letters, make telephone calls

931 *Party Affiliations, e.g., Democratic, Republican, etc.* DD: 329 LC: JK 2311-2359, HX 626-795

The small minority of Americans who are active in political parties exert influence on the political scene far greater than those citizens who merely vote. Party members help select and elect candidates, and influence policy through the type of candidates they support. They have less influence on issues as the typical party organization, Democratic or Republican, pays relatively little attention to issues.

Few people appreciate the amount of effort put out by loyal party members. These include regular attendance at party meetings, which are usually incredibly dull, telephoning and visiting neighbors on behalf of candidates, distributing literature at shopping centers, putting on bumper stickers and car tops, erecting signs, etc. The average party member receives few special favors or rewards for all the work he puts in. He does have trickle-down prestige through the opportunity to meet and talk with prominent political figures upon occasion.

There is a strong camaraderie among old time party members, occasionally marred, however, by intense feuds.

Although candidates rely heavily on resources outside the party, party support (usually delivered in the form of free manpower) is sufficiently important that candidates have to meet the screening criteria of the party. The most important of these is party loyalty, best demonstrated by length of membership, effort expended for the party and strict adherence to party norms and values.

940 Religious Organizations

ENVIRONMENTAL FACTORS: indoor, outdoor, no specific environment, modicum of space, requires little or no equipment, equipment normally at hand.

SOCIAL-PSYCHOLOGICAL FACTORS: aesthetic, utilitarian, pre-patterned, abstract, concrete, group effort, individual effort, structured, supervised, opportunity for recognition.

Impairment Limitations

blind	+	balance	+	*hands impaired:*	1	2
low vision	+	seizures	+	reaching	+	+
hearing	S1	*aphasia:*		handling	+	+
speech	S2	receptive	S3	fingering	+	+
retardation	+	expressive	S3	feeling	+	+
memory	+	mixed	S3	no hands	+	
impaired:						
stooping	+	wheel chair	M1	bed patient	S4	
kneeling	+	semi-ambulant	M1	respiratory	+	
crouching	+	Class III heart	+	*Energy Expenditure in*		
crawling	+	Class IV heart	S4	*METS:* 1.2-3.2		

M1 check access to buildings via ramps and elevators and accessibility of toilet facilities
S1 read religious material instead of listening to services, etc.
S2 can do everything except participate in teaching and discussion groups
S3 will be limited to activities requiring little communication with others
S4 can carry on telephoning activities

941 Formal Church Membership

Formal Church Membership, e.g., Anglican, Baptist, Catholic, Christian Scientist, Jewish, Lutheran, Methodist, Unitarian, etc. DD: 280 LC: BV 820

Formal church membership, for many people, is an almost automatic status starting in childhood. For others, a decision is made to enter formal membership in adulthood. In any event, accepting formal church membership entails entering a cluster of role privileges and obligations. On the privilege side, the member is entitled to the help of the minister for formal ceremonies and in times of illness or death. Informal help, both psychological and material, may be extended by members of the congregation. On the obligation side, members are expected to share the theology, philosophy and ideology of the church, to contribute to the financial burden of supporting the church and, from time to time, to accept special assignments in church activities. Regular attendance at church services is an ideal type role requirement.

950 Cultural and Educational Groups

ENVIRONMENTAL FACTORS: indoor, no specific environment, modicum of space, requires little or no equipment, equipment normally at hand.

SOCIAL-PSYCHOLOGICAL FACTORS: aesthetic, creative, pre-patterned, abstract, group effort, individual effort, structured, unstructured, supervised, unsupervised, opportunity for recognition.

Impairment Limitations

blind	M1	balance	+	*hands impaired:*	*1*	*2*
low vision	M2	seizures	+	reaching	+	+
hearing	0	*aphasia:*		handling	+	+
speech	0	receptive	0	fingering	+	+
retardation	0	expressive	0	feeling	+	+
memory	0	mixed	0	no hands	+	

impaired:

stooping	+	wheel chair	M3	bed patient	0
kneeling	+	semi-ambulant	M3	respiratory	+
crouching	+	Class III heart	+	*Energy Expenditure in*	
crawling	+	Class IV heart	0	*METS:* 1.2-2.3	

M1 braille or talking books
M2 large print
M3 check access to buildings via ramps and elevators and accessibility of toilet facilities

953 *Book Clubs* DD: 374.22 LC: Z 1008, Z 549

A book club is a discussion group which over a period of time develops certain additional dimensions of interpersonal relationships. As book club members come to know each other better, they are able to lower their defenses and say what they really think, a refreshing change from the banality of most day-to-day conversations.

Members frequently belong to one or more of the same organizations as other members, which is an additional thread in making the book club a more cohesive social group than the usual time-limited or topic-limited discussion groups.

960 *Social Groups*

ENVIRONMENTAL FACTORS: indoor, outdoor, no specific environment, modicum of space, equipment a major factor, equipment normally at hand.

SOCIAL-PSYCHOLOGICAL FACTORS: aesthetic, pre-patterned, concrete, group effort, structured, supervised, opportunity for recognition.

Impairment Limitations

blind	M1	balance	S2	*hands impaired:*	*1*	*2*
low vision	M1	seizures	+	reaching	+	M4
hearing	M2	*aphasia:*		handling	+	M4
speech	M2	receptive	M2	fingering	+	M4
retardation	S1	expressive	M2	feeling	+	M4
memory	M3	mixed	M2	no hands	M4	

impaired:

stooping	S3	wheel chair	M5	bed patient	S4
kneeling	S3	semi-ambulant	M5	respiratory	+
crouching	S3	Class III heart	S3	*Energy Expenditure in*	
crawling	S3	Class IV heart	S4	*METS:* 1.2-26.0	

This is a very heterogeneous grouping in terms of physical requirements of the activity. Since the physical requirements have already been indicated on other check list sheets the emphasis here is mainly on communication and social interaction aspects of carrying on activities in groups.

M1 may need companion for travel

M2 may need special sponsoring to be accepted by group

M3 carry notebook with names of the people in the group

M4 may use push button telephones for maintaining organizational contacts by telephone

M5 check access to buildings via ramps & elevators and accessibility of toilet facilities

S1 limit to simple activities with other MR's

S2 exclude athletic and dance activities

S3 exclude some athletic and dance activities

S4 can maintain some organizational contacts by telephone

963 Square Dance Clubs DD: 793.3 LC: GV 1589-1799

A unifying experience for members of square dance clubs is a common set of skills and techniques known and practiced by all members although there are sex variations and variations between the beginners and the old timers. The dance systematically arranges physical contact among every member of a dance square of eight people and since individuals rotate through squares, they are in contact with a substantial number of dancers on any one evening.

Dance clubs travel around, dancing in different dance halls and to different callers. Miscellaneous ritual is developed, including the wearing of distinctive costumes and pins.

967 YMCA, YWCA, YMHA, YWHA DD: 796.5422 LC. BV 1000-1220, BV 1300-1393, DS 101, HS 2226-2230

The Young Men's Christian Association (YMCA) is a middle class organization which provides athletic facilities in the form of gyms and pools, with excellent training and sport programs for both men and boys. For many years, it has been a forerunner in helping middle aged men stay in good physical condition, a movement which is receiving a great deal of current attention. It has also provided dormitory style housing at a reasonable price, which has been valuable for men with limited incomes moving into a city. Diversified educational and social programs are also provided.

The Young Women's Christian Association (YWCA) has provided the same functions for women as the YMCA has for men but, in addition, has become a social change agent frequently on the forefront of promoting improvements in race relations, civic conditions, etc.

The Young Men's Hebrew Association (YMHA) and the Young Women's Hebrew Association (YWHA) offer services similar to those of the YMCA and the YWCA, but with more specific focus on Jewish heritage, culture and special needs.

970 Ethnic Organizations

ENVIRONMENTAL FACTORS: indoor, outdoor, no specific environment, modicum of space, requires little or no equipment, equipment normally at hand.

SOCIAL-PSYCHOLOGICAL FACTORS: aesthetic, creative, pre-patterned, concrete, group effort, individual effort, structured, supervised, opportunity for recognition.

Impairment Limitations

blind	+	balance	+	*hands impaired:*	1	2
low vision	+	seizures	+	reaching	+	+
hearing	M1	*aphasia:*		handling	+	+
speech	M1	receptive	M1	fingering	+	+
retardation	+	expressive	M1	feeling	+	+
memory	M2	mixed	M1	no hands	+	

impaired:

stooping	+	wheel chair	M3	bed patient	S1
kneeling	+	semi-ambulant	M3	respiratory	+
crouching	+	Class III heart	+	*Energy Expenditure in*	
crawling	+	Class IV heart	S1	*METS:* 1.2-4.4	

M1 may need special sponsoring to be accepted by group
M2 carry notebook with names of the people in the group
M3 check access to buildings via ramps and elevators and accessibility of toilet facilities
S1 can maintain some organizational contacts by telephone

970 Ethnic Organizations DD: 301.451, 369 LC: GN

Groups whose unifying factor is a stress on particular ethnic identification can offer perfect opportunities to induce greater social contacts, especially among the elderly. This for two reasons: the elderly are more inclined to identify strongly with a particular ethnic group—a formal organization built around ethnic unification will have immediate appeal; the elderly are more in need of a powerful outside stimulus to encourage social activity—in a sense, they are already part of the group, the requirements are already met by virtue of their being who they are, so it is much easier to consider joining the group if there already exists some element of familiarity. The majority of these ethnic groups are strictly social in nature. No great demands are made of those who join. One grows within the group at one's own pace, comes and goes at will. There is personal and group pride—"I am one of these."

Along with these groups devoted to the perpetration and appreciation of one's own cultural characteristics, there are those organized for the appreciation and experiencing of another's, the groups devoted to international exchange. The appeal of these is somewhat different. Those who desire the protection and nourishment of the familiar may not be attracted by the investigation of the foreign. Some, however, find the prospect fascinating. Some may be familiar with the other's language, or may want to learn it. Some may be interested in the customs, manners and dress without regard for the language. Some may want to share literature or art. Here the strength is more in the individual than from the group. Again, however, participation can encourage social relationships at a self-determined pace.

Finally there are groups which grew out of particular political, economic, or social conditions. They have strong ethnic identifications, as do the first group, but have more pragmatic goals than just socializing, usually because their ethnic group is a minority with lower economic status. They are often quite politically active in the community. They are heavily concerned with the interests of the particular group they represent, and are often a source of controversy to the groups they don't represent. The psychology of groups of this nature is quite different from that of either of the other two groups discussed here. The appeal is to a sense of both individual and group pride and the organization is of a far more utilitarian nature than the types previously mentioned. Involvement in one of these has greater and more emotionally charged implications and most likely the elderly or disabled would not be immediately attracted.

980 Volunteer Service Organizations

ENVIRONMENTAL FACTORS: indoor, outdoor, no specific environment, modicum of space, requires little or no equipment, equipment normally at hand.

SOCIAL-PSYCHOLOGICAL FACTORS: utilitarian, pre-patterned, concrete, group effort, individual effort, structured, supervised, opportunity for recognition.

Impairment Limitations

blind	S1	balance	S2	*hands impaired:*	1	2
low vision	+	seizures	S2	reaching	+	S2
hearing	S2	*aphasia:*		handling	+	S2
speech	+	receptive	S2	fingering	+	S2
retardation	M1	expressive	S2	feeling	+	+
memory	+	mixed	S2	no hands	S2	

impaired:					
stooping	+	wheel chair	S2	bed patient	0
kneeling	+	semi-ambulant	S2	respiratory	S2
crouching	+	Class III heart	S2	*Energy Expenditure in*	
crawling	+	Class IV heart	0	*METS:* 1.2-14.0	

This is a very heterogeneous grouping in terms of the physical requirements of the activity.
M1 may need companion for guidance
S1 could be part of welcoming group or library groups (braille books)
S2 exclude protection groups

983 Educational Groups, e.g., PTA, library groups, etc. DD: 370.1931 LC: LC 230-235

The function of the PTA (Parent-Teachers Association) has varied from community to community. In some, it has been the medium through which the educational philosophy and methods of a school have been explained to the parents. In others, it has been primarily an opportunity for parents to meet teachers in a semi-social situation. It has been used as a springboard for aspiring candidates to attain the visibility necessary to run successfully for a school board office. Partly because of its constitution, the PTA has rarely been effective in exerting pressure for better schools.

Library groups are fortunate in having clear-cut goals: a bigger and better library building, more books and more librarians. Many small town libraries have been started and nourished to adulthood by devoted library groups working over a period of years to raise funds for this cause.

984 Humane Societies, e.g., ASPCA, etc. DD: 364.178 LC: HV 4701-4959

Humane societies have had clear-cut goals—to treat animals in more humane ways. They have not been led astray and frustrated by such irrelevancies as the rank, social class and religion of the animals or whether or not the animals were receiving public welfare instead of earning a living. There have been continuing battles over the use of animals for research purposes.

990 Miscellaneous Organizations (such as fraternities, sororities, professional organizations, toastmasters' clubs)

ENVIRONMENTAL FACTORS: indoor, no specific environment, modicum of space, requires little or no equipment, equipment normally at hand.

SOCIAL-PSYCHOLOGICAL FACTORS: aesthetic, utilitarian, pre-patterned, abstract, concrete, group effort, structured, supervised, opportunity for recognition.

Impairment Limitations

						hands impaired:	*1*	*2*
blind	+	balance	+			reaching	+	+
low vision	+	seizures	+			handling	+	+
hearing	S1	*aphasia:*				fingering	+	+
speech	S1	receptive	S1, 2			feeling	+	+
retardation	S1, S2	expressive	S1, 2			no hands	+	
memory	S1	mixed	S1, 2					

impaired:

stooping	+	wheel chair	+	bed patient	S3
kneeling	+	semi-ambulant	+	respiratory	+
crouching	+	Class III heart	+	*Energy Expenditure in*	
crawling	+	Class IV heart	S3	*METS:* 1.2-4.4	

S1 exclude toastmaster's club
S2 exclude honor societies, college fraternities and sororities, professional organizations
S3 may maintain some organizational contacts by telephone
M1 check access to buildings via ramp and elevators and suitable toilet facilities

991 Honor Societies DD: 371.852 LC: LB 3602

Academic honor societies serve a dual purpose: they allow the academic community to recognize and encourage intellectual achievements, and they allow the members of the society to make social contacts with others of similar intellectual capabilities. Both of these functions are important, the second extremely so.

The adolescent who excels intellectually often finds himself rejected by the majority of his peer group, especially if he tends to be introverted and does not possess exceptional leadership ability or athletic talents. In an honor society, this type of student can find others who share his interests, with whom he can be open without fear of ridicule, and he can sharpen his wits through discussion and debate with others of high intellectual capabilities.

Almost conversely, for the high achiever with an overdeveloped ego, an honor society can be humbling. The eight-day wonder suddenly finds himself with a group who will not automatically or even quickly acknowledge his superiority and among whom he may not even *be* superior. Although this kind of experience may be frightening at first, it can be very helpful in terms of establishing perspective about capabilities and roles in society.

Although there is undeniably a certain amount of intellectual snobbery connected with honor societies, the main thrust, at least within the society, tends to be democratic. The superior individual finds a peer group, among whom he is no longer superior; no matter what the social standing of various members of the society, all come together as equals or near-equals in the intellectual quest.

Academic honor societies function chiefly through high schools and colleges, although college groups, especially, may have active graduate or alumni branches. Honor societies often engage in service projects, which give the members opportunities to work together. Tutoring underprivileged youth is a favorite project in these socially-conscious times.

An exception to the school-oriented nature of these groups is the organization called Mensa, an international association whose sole criterion for admission is very high intelligence. In addition to providing a meeting ground for people of high intellectual calibre (members often collaborate on projects or use each other as resource people), Mensa considers one of its chief purposes to be providing a homogeneously high-intelligence group to be available for research of various types.

992 *Investment Clubs* DD: 332.6 LC: HG 4530

Members of an investment club are drawn together by the fascination of trying to make money through investments. They are dependent upon each other because the capital of any one individual is usually not large enough to permit any diversification of funds, whereas the pooled capital of all the members may make this feasible. It is essentially a form of gambling in which the members of the group are united against an outside opponent, the vagaries of the stock market, rather than being pitted against each other as in a poker club. This makes it a desirable activity for individuals who enjoy gambling but do not enjoy competition against friends.

995 *Organizations for the Handicapped, e.g., the paraplegia association* DD: 361-362 LC: LC 1041-7, HV 1-4959

Members of these organizations are closely drawn together by their common impairment.Whether they were impaired genetically, at birth, in early childhood or not until recently will make a substantial difference in their identification with the organization including sometimes a considerable resentment of it. Unlike the identity-seeking of minority groups and Women's Liberation, as yet there does not seem to have arisen among these groups any publically proclaimed positive identity. There are no announced claims to positive virtues such as "because we have suffered we have more insight" or "because we need more help ourselves we offer more help to our fellow members" or "because we cannot get around we are able to devote more time to such valuable activities as reading, writing, arts, crafts and music." Except for the organizations for the blind, the organizations themselves generate little public demand for better opportunities for their members.

QUICK FIND LIST

ENVIRONMENTAL FACTORS

Indoor			Outdoor		No specific environment			Specialized environment and/or climate
112	390	680	112	390	112	430	710	222
120	410	690	170	440	120	450	720	224
130	430	710	210	480	130	460	740	227
140	450	720	221	580	140	470	750	228
150	460	740	222	590	150	480	760	233
160	470	750	224	610	160	510	770	264
170	480	770	225	620	190	520	780	290
190	510	780	226	630	210	530	790	320
210	520	790	227	640	221	540	810	340
225	530	810	228	660	225	550	820	350
226	540	820	232	670	226	560	830	370
227	550	830	233	680	232	570	880	380
232	560	880	241	690	241	580	890	390
241	570	890	242	750	242	590	930	440
242	580	930	247	760	247	620	940	610
247	590	940	256	780	256	630	950	640
256	610	950	262	790	262	640	960	780
262	620	960	264	830	274	650	970	790
264	630	970	274	840	310	660	980	840
290	640	980	290	880	380	670	990	890
310	650	990	310	890	390	680		
370	660		320	930	410	690		
380	670		340	940				
			350	960				
			370	970				
			380	980				

Modicum of space			Unlimited space	Requires little or no equipment		Equipment a major factor	
120	430	680	112	112	630	120	510
130	450	690	170	140	640	130	520
140	460	710	221	150	650	170	530
150	470	720	222	160	660	190	540
160	480	740	224	210	680	221	550
170	510	750	225	225	740	222	560
190	520	770	226	227	750	224	570
210	530	780	227	241	760	225	580
232	540	790	228	242	770	226	590
241	550	810	233	247	780	227	610
242	560	820	274	249	790	228	620
247	570	830	320	256	810	232	640
256	580	880	340	274	830	233	670
262	590	890	350	310	930	262	690
264	610	930	370	320	940	264	710
290	620	940	380	370	950	290	720
310	630	950	390	390	970	340	750
370	640	960	440	410	980	350	780
380	650	970	590	430	990	370	790
390	660	980	660	440		380	820
410	670	990	760			390	840
			780			450	880
			840			460	890
			890			470	
						480	960

ENVIRONMENTAL FACTORS

Equipment normally at hand				Equipment not necessarily at hand						
140	430	720	830	112	222	241	340	460	580	670
150	440	740	890	120	224	242	350	470	590	690
210	510	750	930	130	226	247	370	480	610	750
225	520	760	940	160	227	256	380	530	620	780
274	550	770	950	170	228	262	390	540	630	790
310	650	780	960	190	232	264	410	560	640	840
320	660	790	970	221	233	290	450	570	650	880
370	680	810	980							
390	710	820	990							

SOCIAL-PSYCHOLOGICAL FACTORS

Aesthetic			Utilitarian		Creative		Pre-patterned		
112	274	610	120	710	130	560	112	310	710
120	290	620	190	720	150	570	120	320	720
130	310	630	256	740	170	590	130	340	740
140	320	640	350	780	190	610	140	380	750
150	340	650	370	790	221	620	150	390	760
160	350	660	380	810	222	630	160	410	770
170	370	670	390	820	225	640	170	430	780
190	380	680	480	830	227	650	190	450	790
210	390	690	510	840	228	660	210	460	810
221	410	710	520	880	340	670	224	470	820
222	430	720	530	890	350	680	226	480	830
224	440	740	550	930	370	690	232	510	840
225	450	750	560	940	380	760	233	530	880
226	460	760	570	980	390	780	241	540	890
227	470	770	580	990	440	790	242	560	930
228	480	780	620		510	810	247	570	940
232	510	790			520	930	256	580	950
233	520	930			530	950	262	620	960
241	530	940			550	970	264	650	970
242	540	950					274	660	980
247	550	960					290	670	990
256	560	970							
262	570	990							
264	590								

Avocational Activities for the Handicapped

SOCIAL-PSYCHOLOGICAL FACTORS

Abstract	Concrete			Group Effort		Individual Effort		
130	112	290	610	112	510	112	340	650
140	120	310	620	140	530	120	350	660
150	130	320	640	150	610	130	370	670
190	140	340	660	160	650	140	380	680
390	160	350	670	190	660	150	390	690
470	170	370	680	221	670	160	410	710
480	190	380	710	222	690	170	430	720
610	210	390	720	226	760	190	440	740
630	221	410	760	227	770	210	450	750
650	222	430	780	228	780	221	460	760
670	224	440	790	232	790	222	470	770
680	225	450	810	233	840	224	480	780
690	226	460	820	241	880	225	510	790
710	227	470	830	242	890	226	520	810
740	228	480	840	247	930	227	530	820
750	232	510	880	262	940	228	540	830
770	233	520	890	264	950	233	550	840
810	241	530	930	290	960	241	560	880
930	242	540	940	320	970	242	570	890
940	247	550	960	340	980	247	580	930
950	256	560	970	380	990	256	590	940
990	262	570	980	390		274	610	950
	264	580	990	450		290	620	970
	274	590				310	630	980
						320	640	

Structured			Unstructured		Supervised		Unsupervised		
112	274	750	150	520	120	670	112	380	580
120	290	760	190	550	130	710	160	390	590
130	390	770	221	560	140	720	170	410	610
140	430	780	222	570	150	750	190	430	620
150	450	790	224	590	222	760	210	440	630
160	460	810	225	610	227	770	221	450	640
170	470	820	226	620	232	780	222	460	650
190	510	830	227	630	233	790	224	470	660
210	530	840	228	640	241	810	225	480	670
231	540	880	310	650	242	820	226	510	680
232	580	890	320	660	247	830	227	520	690
233	620	930	340	670	256	840	228	530	740
241	650	940	350	680	262	880	310	540	760
242	660	950	370	690	264	890	320	550	780
247	670	960	380	740	274	930	340	560	790
256	680	970	390	760	290	940	350	570	950
262	710	980	410	780	340	950	370		
264	720	990	440	790	390	960			
			480	950	570	970			
					650	980			
					660	990			

SOCIAL-PSYCHOLOGICAL FACTORS

Opportunity for recognition				Little opportunity for recognition	
112	264	540	760	160	380
120	274	550	770	190	390
130	290	560	780	210	410
140	350	570	790	221	430
150	370	580	810	222	670
170	380	590	840	224	710
225	390	610	880	225	720
227	440	620	890	226	740
232	450	630	930	227	750
233	460	640	940	228	760
241	470	650	950	310	780
242	480	660	960	320	790
247	510	670	970	340	820
256	520	680	980	370	830
262	530	690	990		

IMPAIRMENT LIMITATIONS

blind			low vision			hearing		
+	S	M	+	S	M	+	S	M
640	160	112	130	210	112	112	440	290	150
640	160	112	130	210	112	112	440	290	150
670	210	130	150	221	120	120	450	650	210
710	310	140	160	310	140	130	460	750	221
930	350	150	170	350	222	140	470	790	320
940	370	190	190	540	224	160	480	810	390
970	470	222	274	580	225	170	510	820	720
990	480	224	380	590	226	190	520	830	960
	540	225	410	610	227	222	530	930	970
	550	226	450	650	228	224	540	940	
	580	227	460	740	256	225	550	980	
	610	228	470	750	320	226	560	990	
	650	256	480	780	340	227	570		
	740	320	520	810	370	228	580		
	750	340	530	820	390	232	590		
	780	370	550	840	430	233	610		
	810	380	640		510	241	620		
	820	390	660		560	242	630		
	980	510	670		570	247	640		
		530	680		620	256	660		
		560	710		630	262	680		
		570	720		950	264	690		
		660	760		960	274	740		
		680	770			310	760		
		720	790			340	770		
		760	830			350	780		
		770	930			370	840		
		790	940			380	880		
		950	970			410	890		
		960	980			430			
			990						

IMPAIRMENT LIMITATIONS

		speech					*retardation*		
	+		S	M		+		S	M
112	290	610	650	150	112	274	560	160	130
120	310	620	790	850	120	290	570	190	140
130	320	630	810	860	170	310	590	580	150
140	340	640	820	960	210	320	610	620	340
160	350	660	930	970	221	350	630	780	760
170	370	670	940		222	370	640	790	980
190	380	680	990		224	380	650	930	
210	390	690			225	410	660	960	
221	410	710			226	430	670	990	
222	430	720			227	440	710		
224	440	740			228	450	720		
225	450	750			232	460	750		
226	460	760			233	470	770		
227	470	770			241	480	830		
228	480	780			242	510	840		
232	510	830			247	520	880		
233	520	840			256	530	940		
241	530	880			262	540	970		
242	540	890			264	550			
247	550	980							
256	560								
262	570								
264	580								
274	590								

IMPAIRMENT LIMITATIONS

Memory +		S	M		Balance +		S	M
112	520	160	130	440	130	560	112	120
120	530	190	140	450	140	620	170	222
170	540	780	150	470	150	630	320	227
210	550	790	221	510	160	640	350	231
225	560	830	222	580	190	650	370	380
228	570	930	224	610	210	670	520	510
232	590	990	226	660	310	680	590	570
233	620		227	670	340	710	780	580
242	630		241	690	390	720	830	610
256	640		247	760	410	740	890	690
264	680		262	790	430	750	960	760
274	710		320	840	440	770	980	790
290	720		340	960	450	810		840
310	740		410	970	460	820		880
350	750		430		470	870		
370	770				480	930		
380	880				530	940		
460	940				540	950		
480	980				550	970		
						990		

IMPAIRMENT LIMITATIONS

Seizures +			S	M	Aphasia: Receptive +			S	M
112	390	660	225	370	112	262	540	160	130
120	410	670	290	380	120	264	550	190	150
130	430	680	320	510	140	274	560	290	210
140	440	690	350	570	170	310	570	510	340
150	450	710	520	580	221	320	590	580	670
160	460	720	780	590	222	350	610	780	760
170	470	740	830	760	224	370	620	790	960
190	480	750	890	790	225	380	630	840	970
210	530	770	980	840	226	410	640	930	
232	540	810		880	227	430	660	940	
233	550	820			228	440	690	980	
241	560	930			232	450	710	990	
242	610	940			233	460	720		
247	620	950			241	470	750		
262	630	960			242	480	770		
274	640	970			247	520	880		
310	650	990			256	530			
340									

IMPAIRMENT LIMITATIONS

	Aphasia:	*Expressive*				*Aphasia:*	*Mixed*		
	+		S	M		+		S	M
112	264	550	160	150	112	262	540	160	130
120	274	560	190	390	120	264	550	190	210
130	290	570	650	760	140	274	560	290	340
140	310	580	790	960	170	310	570	510	760
170	320	590	830	970	221	320	590	580	960
210	340	610	840		222	350	610	780	970
221	350	620	930		224	370	620	790	
222	370	630	940		225	380	630	840	
224	380	640	980		226	410	640	930	
225	410	660	990		227	430	660	940	
226	430	670			228	440	670	980	
227	440	690			232	450	690	990	
228	450	710			233	460	710		
232	460	720			241	470	720		
233	470	740			242	480	750		
241	480	750			247	520	770		
242	510	770			256	530	880		
247	520	780							
256	530	880							
262	540								

IMPAIRMENT LIMITATIONS

	Reaching (one hand impaired)				*Reaching (two hands impaired)*			
	+		S	M	+		S	M
112	380	720	221	120	210	710	190	130
130	390	740	222	140	224	720	225	140
150	410	750	228	170	274	740	228	150
160	430	760	530	247	310	750	370	160
190	440	770	580	262	320	760	580	226
210	450	780	650	264	410	770	590	340
224	460	790	660	510	430	790	650	350
225	470	810	670	520	450	930	660	390
226	480	840	820	550	460	940	670	510
227	540	880	830	570	470	950	810	520
232	560	890		610	480	970	820	550
241	590	930			540	990	830	560
242	620	940			620		890	570
274	630	950			680		980	610
310	640	960						630
320	680	970						780
340	690	980						880
350	710	990						960
370								

IMPAIRMENT LIMITATIONS

Handling (one hand impaired)		+		S	M	Handling (two hands impaired)		
						+	S	M
112	370	740	221	120		210	190	130
130	380	750	222	140		274	225	140
150	390	760	227	170		310	227	150
160	410	770	228	247		320	228	160
190	430	780	640	262		460	590	226
210	440	790	650	264		660	650	340
224	450	810	670	510		750	670	390
225	460	840	820	520		760	810	470
226	470	880	830	530		770	820	480
232	480	890		540		930	830	510
241	590	930		550		940	890	550
242	630	940		560		950	980	570
274	660	950		570		970		580
310	680	960		580		990		620
320	690	970		610				630
340	710	980		620				680
350	720	990						710
								720
								740
								780
								790
								880
								960

IMPAIRMENT LIMITATIONS

Fingering (one hand impaired)					Fingering (two hands impaired)		
+			S	M	+	S	M
112	340	720	221	120	210	190	120
130	350	740	222	140	241	225	130
150	370	750	227	170	242	227	140
160	380	760	228	247	262	228	150
190	390	770	640	510	264	380	160
210	410	780	650	520	274	590	226
224	430	790	670	530	290	650	340
225	440	810	820	540	310	670	390
226	450	840	830	550	320	810	470
232	460	880		560	460	820	480
233	470	890		570	660	830	510
241	480	930		580	750	890	550
242	590	940		610	760	980	570
262	630	950		620	770		580
264	660	960			930		620
274	680	970			940		630
290	690	980			950		680
310	710	990			970		710
320	710				990		720
							740
							780
							790
							880
							960

IMPAIRMENT LIMITATIONS

Feeling (one hand impaired)					Feeling (two hands impaired)					No hands		
+			S	M	+			S	M	+	S	M
112	320	660	221	120	130	370	660	190	120	210	190	130
130	340	680	227	510	140	390	690	225	340	274	225	140
140	350	690	228	570	150	410	710	227	450	310	228	150
150	370	710	670	580	160	430	720	228	510	320	650	160
160	380	720		590	210	440	740	320	570	750	660	226
170	390	740		780	222	460	750	380	580	760	670	340
190	410	750		830	226	470	760	670	590	770	810	390
210	430	760		840	241	480	770	810	640	930	820	470
222	440	770			242	520	790	820	680	940	890	480
224	450	790			247	530	890		780	950	980	510
225	460	810			262	540	930		830	970		550
226	470	820			264	550	940		840	990		580
232	480	880			274	610	950		880			620
233	520	890			290	620	970		960			630
241	530	930			310	630	980					680
242	540	940			350	650	990					710
247	550	950										720
262	610	960										740
264	620	970										780
274	630	980										790
290	640	990										880
310	650											960

IMPAIRMENT LIMITATIONS

	Impaired Stooping					*Impaired Kneeling*			
	+		S	M		+		S	M
130	540	740	170	112	130	450	680	170	112
140	550	750	221	120	140	460	710	221	120
150	560	760	222	274	150	470	720	225	274
160	570	770	225	340	160	480	740	227	340
190	590	790	227	380	190	520	750	320	510
210	610	810	320	510	210	530	760	350	690
224	620	820	350	690	222	540	770	370	780
310	630	830	370	780	224	550	790	390	840
410	640	890	390	840	232	560	810	440	
430	650	930	440		233	570	820	580	
450	660	940	580		241	590	830	880	
460	670	950	880		242	610	890	960	
470	680	970	960		247	620	930		
480	710	980			262	630	940		
520	720	990			290	640	950		
530					310	650	970		
					380	660	980		
					410	670	990		
					430				

IMPAIRMENT LIMITATIONS

Impaired Crouching					Impaired Crawling				
+			S	M	+			S	M
130	530	740	170	112	112	380	660	221	274
140	540	750	221	120	120	410	670	225	690
150	550	760	222	274	130	430	680	227	780
160	560	770	225	340	140	440	710	228	
190	570	790	227	380	150	450	720	320	
210	590	810	320	510	160	460	740	350	
224	610	820	350	690	170	470	750	370	
242	620	830	370	780	190	480	760	390	
310	630	890	390	840	210	510	770	580	
410	640	930	440		222	520	790	880	
430	650	940	580		224	530	810	960	
450	660	950	880		232	540	820		
460	670	970	960		233	550	830		
470	680	980			241	560	840		
480	710	990			242	570	890		
520	720				247	590	930		
					262	610	940		
					264	620	950		
					290	630	970		
					310	640	980		
					340	650	990		

Wheel Chair				Semi-ambulant				Class III heart				
+		S	M	+		S	M	+			S	M
130	540	170	112	130	550	112	120	130	470	720	222	120
140	550	225	120	140	560	170	222	140	480	740	320	232
150	560	227	222	150	620	225	242	150	520	750	350	340
160	610	320	241	160	630	227	340	160	530	760	590	390
190	620	350	242	190	640	320	380	170	540	770	780	440
210	630	370	262	210	650	350	510	190	550	790	960	510
232	640	580	340	310	670	370	520	210	560	810	980	570
310	650	590	380	390	680	580	570	242	610	820		580
390	670	780	510	410	710	590	610	310	620	830		650
410	680	880	520	430	720	780	690	370	630	890		660
430	690	890	570	450	740	880	750	380	640	930		880
450	710	980	750	460	760	890	770	410	670	940		
460	720		760	470	810	980	790	430	680	950		
470	740		770	480	820		930	450	690	970		
480	810		790	530	990		940	460	710	990		
530	820		930	540			950					
	990		940				960					
			950				970					
			960									
			970									

IMPAIRMENT LIMITATIONS

Class IV heart			Bed patient			Respiratory				
+	S	M	+	S	M	+			S	M
130	170	120	130	170	120	130	460	720	320	120
140	390	380	140	225	310	140	470	740	670	226
150	610	520	150	370	380	150	480	750	780	232
160	640	590	160	390	520	160	520	760	980	340
190	650	650	190	590	570	170	530	770		370
210	670		210	610		190	540	790		390
310	770		410	640		210	550	810		440
410	780		430	650		222	560	820		510
430	930		450	670		242	590	830		570
450	940		460	770		310	620	840		580
460	960		470	780		350	630	890		610
470	970		480	820		380	650	930		640
480	990		530	930		410	680	940		660
530			540	940		430	690	950		880
540			550	960		450	710	960		
550			560	970				970		
560			620	990				990		
620			630							
630			680							
680			710							
710			720							
720			740							
740			750							

IMPAIRMENT LIMITATIONS

Energy expenditure in METS

1 - 1.5		1.5 - 2.7			2.7 - 4			4 - 6.6		Over 6.6	
410	710	120	450	750	120	380	770	112	520	112	370
440	720	130	460	760	170	390	780	120	570	221	380
470	740	140	520	770	210	440	790	221	580	224	390
480	750	150	530	780	221	510	810	224	590	225	570
520	760	160	540	790	222	520	820	225	610	227	580
530	770	170	550	810	224	570	830	226	640	228	590
540	780	190	560	820	225	580	840	227	660	247	660
550	790	210	570	830	228	590	880	228	760	256	780
560	810	222	580	880	232	610	890	232	780	262	880
570	820	310	590	890	242	620	930	233	830	264	960
590	830	320	610	930	290	630	940	241	840	274	980
610	930	340	620	940	310	640	960	290	880	290	
620	940	350	630	950	320	650	970	320	890	320	
630	950	370	640	960	340	690	980	340	930		
640	960	380	650	970	350	750	990	350	960		
650	970	390	670	980	370	760		370	970		
680	980	430	690	990				380	980		
690	990	440						390	990		
								440			

INDEX